Living with Osteogenesis Imperfecta

A Guidebook for Families

Edited by
Heidi C. Glauser

Published by
The Osteogenesis Imperfecta Foundation, Inc.

With the release of this first edition, it is anticipated that readers may wish to send corrections or suggestions for future release. The Publisher specifically is interested in expanding the 'Additional Resources Listing' found in Appendix E. All correspondence and inquiries should be directed to:

Family Guidebook.
The Osteogenesis Imprefecta Foundation, Inc.
5005 W. Laurel St., Ste 210
Tampa, FL 33607

ISBN 0-9642189-0-9

**Major Funding for this project
has been provided by
The American Legion
Child Welfare Foundation**

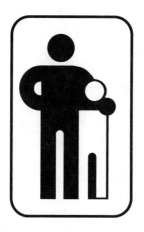

Partial funding for this project
courtesy of the Athwin Foundation

This book is dedicated to
all people with osteogenesis imperfecta
and those who love and work with them.

Acknowledgements

I am grateful to the many people with OI, and parents of children with OI who have contributed to this book through their words and life examples. Special thanks are due to the following people who generously contributed their time, resources, and abilities to the creation of this book. Thanks to Mr. Terry L. Woodburn and the American Legion Child Welfare Foundation, Inc. for initially recognizing the significance of this work, and for their expression of confidence through the provision of major funding for this first-of-its-kind project; to the Athwin Foundation for their funding partnership in support of this project; to Shannon Smith, an intelligent, conscientious, and committed intern, from Pittsburgh, PA, who contributed many hours of research and text processing, and who fulfilled a myriad of assorted assignments to make this book a reality. Thanks to Peter Byers, M.D., Jean Jasinski, Barbara Everson, Chuck Glauser, and Pat Kipperman for their painstaking duties as proof-readers. Thanks to Laura Vinchesi, Smilen Savov, Becky Kronk, Jay Shapiro, M.D., Larry Lawfer, and many others for their contributions of accomplished photography; to Brian Young for his skillful line drawings; to Doug Lathrop for initially getting the project off the ground; to Vonnie Coleman, Executive Director, Osteogenesis Imperfecta Foundation, and my sons, Rhett, Trevor, and Burk for their untiring direct and moral support; and especially to all the authors and consultants who contributed their time, skills, and expertise to the content of this book. And a very special thanks to my buddy and son with OI, Trey, who has been the inspiration behind my years of service to families whose lives are touched by OI.

— *Heidi C. Glauser*

Introduction

I suppose I have known I would work on this book for twelve years, ever since I went looking for a book about osteogenesis imperfecta and could not find it. In 1982 my husband and I were stunned and bewildered parents when our son, Trey, was born with osteogenesis imperfecta. Our search revealed very little information on what to expect, or where to look for help. Although our need was great, we soon realized that the one critical resource we needed was simply unavailable.

Through the Osteogenesis Imperfecta Foundation, (OIF), and years of direct contact with hundreds of people with osteogenesis imperfecta, (OI), one thing is clear; families of children with OI and affected adults crave information about their disorder. They've learned that very little information exists for families except through the Osteogenesis Imperfecta Foundation. Most medical textbooks contain a very short, and sometimes inaccurate, description of OI. These abbreviated depictions or hurried explanations from well-meaning physicians are rarely sufficient to answer the myriad of questions that arise when one lives each day with brittle bones. By the hundreds, families flock to the family support groups and conferences sponsored by OIF. People with OI and their caregivers hunger for information. They yearn to assimilate information from *knowledgeable* professionals and *experienced* peers.

People with osteogenesis imperfecta and their parents, learn early the necessity of becoming advocates for their own, or their child's health care. Especially as physicians become more specialized, it becomes imperative that the person with OI assume an active advocate role. For these reasons, it is important to have a clear understanding of the causes, methods of treatment, social implications, and practical life skills involved in living with OI. Passive dependence on the physician is, in many cases, unacceptable to people with OI.

The mission of the Osteogenesis Imperfecta Foundation is to improve the quality of life for people with osteogenesis imperfecta. Through the support of the Osteogenesis Imperfecta Foundation, the American Legion Child Welfare Foundation, and the Athwin Foundation, this book is fulfilling that goal. It is meant to aid you in recognizing the significance of your symptoms and in effectively managing them as an integral and essential part of your own health care team.

As you leaf through the pages that follow, assume that you are in the presence of a myriad of unhurried doctors and experienced lay people with a broad knowledge of OI. Imagine that the authors of this book have pulled up a chair to chat. We know you will benefit from this broad spectrum of knowledge written in everyday language. The insightful authors have shared methods and treatments to aid you in improving the quality of your life with OI. It is my hope that by sharing our knowledge and strengths together, our lives with OI will be less fragile.

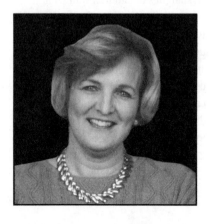

Heidi C. Glauser

Contents

Part I - Medical Issues

Part II - Educational and Social Concerns

Part III - The Day to Day Guide of Living with OI

Appendices

Chapter 1

OI – The Basics

by Peter Bullough, M.D.
Hospital for Special Surgery, New York

Osteo – Bone
Genesis – Formation
Imperfecta – Imperfect

The term osteogenesis imperfecta literally means "bone that is imperfectly made from the beginning of life." Our bodies consist of several hundred bones, all articulating one with another, making it possible for us to move about. If people did not have bones, they would be nothing more than blobs of protoplasm oozing their way across the surface of the earth. Bones make it possible for people to walk, to run, to sit, to enjoy themselves playing games and to do all sorts of activities that would otherwise be impossible.

The human body produces bone all the time. Over a period of ten years, people replace all the bone in their bodies. When looking at normal bone on an X-ray, we see material made up of many plates with a thick skin on the surface. Most of bone, however, is just space - empty of bony calcified tissue. Fat and hematopoietic tissue, which make red blood cells, fill the empty space. The bones are part of the organ system that we call the connective tissue. Connective tissue may be regarded as an organ that pervades the entire body and that is subject to diseases of its own. The connective tissue is like the fabric of the body. Like any other fabric, the connective tissue is constructed of numerous minute threads with filler cement material between.

Most of the organs in the body such as the liver, brain, lungs, and kidneys, are constituted of 99% cells. The connective tissue also contains cells, but here the cells constitute only five percent of the volume. Most of the volume of the tissue is taken up by what is called extracellular matrix. The most important part of the extracellular matrix, the threads of the fabric, is called collagen.

Collagen

Collagen is much like cotton fabric. It is made up of threads which, when woven together into something, resist tensile, or pulling forces. It looks very much like the material of a shirt. If the fabric of your shirt is pulled, it does not rip apart because the weave of the threads holds it together. In the bone, the spaces between the collagen fibers are filled with a hard material that will resist compression. This chalk-like material is a calcium salt called apatite.

Collagen is a protein, and like all the proteins in the body, it is produced by the cells. The information which tells the cell how to make the protein is contained in the cell's chromosomes, or the genes, the material that characterizes you as a human being rather than some other creature. The gene responsible for production of collagen is very complex and has many different pieces of information on it, much like a micro-chip in a computer. It has the ability to replicate itself and send that information to make collagen molecules. If the message is incorrect, as it is in people with OI, the cell cannot make a proper collagen molecule.

Inside the body, all collagen-making cells have to move around in very complicated ways. Currently, we have no idea how that movement is controlled. In such a complicated activity as collagen-making, many things can go wrong. In some cases of OI, the gene that tells the cell how to weave the collagen threads correctly is defective. If a person has a gene that is defective, he or she cannot make collagen properly. We know that to be true for some people with OI.

Collagen-making can be compared to when a cook bakes a cake. If the cook forgets to put in the baking powder, the cake is a disaster. If he puts in only half as much as he should, the cake tastes heavy. And if he puts in too much baking powder, he then must spend the next week cleaning the oven. It is the same with bone formation. There are many things that can go wrong in the recipe. For bone to be exactly right, it needs exactly the right amount and quality of collagen.

Bones

In normal bone, cells are few and far between. It may surprise you to know that there are many more cells in OI bone than in normal bone. This is because the amount of collagen produced by each cell is less than normal. Consequently, the cells are closer together and the overall size of the bone is reduced.

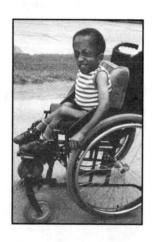

Bone formation in OI can be likened to the following example: imagine three workers on a construction site. One very muscular worker can build a piece of wall measuring ten feet by ten feet, another can make a piece of wall that measures five feet by ten feet, and the third frail worker can only make a piece that measures two feet by ten feet. The three workers are each capable of building various and unequal sizes of structures. The matrix of the bone in OI is like a worker who cannot build a large enough section of wall; it makes less collagen than a normal cell makes and because of this, the resulting product is smaller and weaker.

The difference between a man who is seven feet tall and one who is four feet ten inches is not in the number of cells he has. The person who is seven feet tall simply makes a bigger package of collagen, and, therefore, his skeleton is much bigger than a person who is four feet tall. The shorter person makes a smaller package of collagen. People with OI make a very small package of collagen, so small that they do not have enough to hold the system together very well.

Classification of OI

It is generally accepted that OI is not one disorder but rather a whole set of disorders. It was originally thought that there were just two types of OI. Those with mild OI were called OI tarda, or meaning late or "not seen at birth". Those with the more severe clinical disorder were referred to as OI congenita, or "seen at birth". From a practical, clinical standpoint this is true. Yet, it has become very clear that an extremely wide variance of symptoms and manifestations exists in people who have OI. OI is not simply one or even two disorders. There are at least four main types of OI as represented on the figures 1-1 and 1-2. In addition to these four types, sub-classifications are being developed as we study X-rays and collagen further.

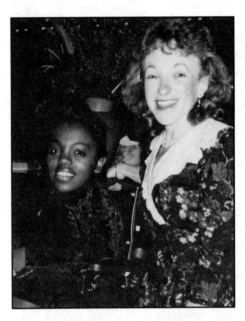

Incidence of OI

The incidence of OI is consistent throughout the world. In other words, the number of people with OI per 100,000 of the population, is just as great in the United States as it is in China or Sweden. OI does not affect any race or ethnic group more than another. Although no one knows for sure, it is estimated that the overall frequency for OI identifiable at birth is about 1 in 20,000 to 30,000.[4] OI Type I, the mildest form, occurs most frequently. It is estimated that the remaining types, II, III, and IV each occur at approximately the same rate.[5] Since people with the milder forms sometimes are not aware they have OI, it is difficult to account for the full population of people who have OI, and actual OI incidence remains uncertain. Because many of the babies born with severe OI rarely live, the incidence of OI in the newborn population is higher than those who are now alive.

Clinical Features of OI

Fractures

OI is characterized by bones that break easily. This is partly because the amount and strength of bone is insufficient to hold up the weight of a person or to resist the force put on the bone when a muscle is contracted. Normal bone is able to withstand most falls. But if a person with OI has even a minor accident, the bones can break. It is possible for people with OI to break a bone without being aware of the fracture, but generally, and especially with fractures of the large bones, the pain associated with a fracture is severe and the ensuing deformity prevents normal function.

The bones in the spine are apt to break without the person realizing it. People with OI almost always have curvature in the spine. This curvature, or scoliosis, results from the accumulation of small fractures which gradually deform the spine.

Deformities

In severe OI, the accumulation of fractures can lead to noticeable deformities in the bone. Each time a bone is broken and set it will heal in a position that is slightly less than perfect. After 30 or 40 fractures the bone will be noticeably bent. Problems with deformity occur particularly in the limbs and spine. There are some people who have had very few fractures but who experience marked deformity. Usually this is because the muscles are stronger than the OI bone and the bone gradually changes in shape.

Stature

People with OI often are extremely short statured. At the end of every bone there is a plate of cartilage where all growth in bone length occurs from birth until age 16. In the unaffected population, the plate of cartilage is very well protected and supported by bone on either side of it. In OI, where there is a great deficiency in bone, the growth plate may fracture or actually crumple, just as the bone itself fractures. Accumulation of fractures in the growth plates may affect the ability of the bone to grow to its full length. Because of this, most people with OI, except for the milder cases, are short-statured to varying degrees.

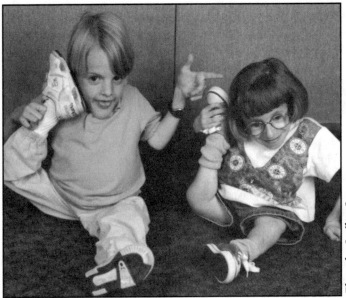

Photo by Smilen Savov

Skin and Joints

The skin layer of many people with OI tends to be thin because of the poor collagen underneath the skin. Also, the ligaments or tendons are not very strong. Many children with OI enjoy impressing their friends with the laxity of their joints, yet this laxity can lead to difficulties in the stability of the ankles and other joints.

Sclerae

A blue hue to the sclerae, or whites of the eyes, is a common feature in OI. This hue is due, in part, to this thin layer of skin as mentioned above. Blue sclerae is present in some families, not in others, and in some families, over time it has been known to fade to a pale blue or white.

Teeth

Poor collagen is the reason people with OI often have problems with their teeth. The enamel, or outer layer of the tooth, which normally makes teeth look white, can crumple and wear away in OI.

This is because the underlying dentin is abnormal. Although there is usually no pain or sensitivity in the teeth, the exposed underlying dentin gets stained and appears brownish or grey. This soft dentin can rapidly wear away, leaving the visible portion of the teeth almost gone. The resulting problem is in the appearance and function of the teeth.

Hearing Impairment

In OI Type I, hearing loss affects many of adults to some degree by the age of 50, although it is rarely a problem before the age of ten. Hearing impairment is much less common in OI Type III and IV.[6] Tiny fractures in the bones of the inner ear can occur and affect the hearing of people with OI. It is advised that people with OI refrain from exposure to loud sounds resulting from sources such as loud music or from occupational sources.

Muscles

A fracture in a person with OI is followed by a period of immobilization in which the musculature in the limb atrophies. And because the person does not develop the musculature, the bone also does not develop as it should. In order to form strong bones, the bones must receive constant stress.

A tennis player knows that the arm used to swing the racket generally has better developed muscles compared with the other arm. If an X-ray of that arm was taken, it would be evident that the bone underneath was thicker too. The bone is thicker because muscle development is greater. The contractions in the thicker muscle put more stress on the bone, and that action thickens the bone.

Bone development is very dependent upon muscle development. This is the reason why women are strongly advised to get regular exercise to prevent osteoporosis. Similarly, in OI, people need to develop their musculature to its maximum potential. Since they have so little muscle to begin with, they must exercise to the maximum in order to thicken and strengthen their muscles and bones as much as possible.

Thinning of the Bone

OI is associated with thinning of the bone. The thinning of the bone increases the risk of fractures. A person who has fractured a bone knows that when the limb comes out of the cast six weeks afterwards, the muscles have shrunk. It generally takes a full year to build up the shrunken muscle to what it was before. Upon X-raying the bone after a fracture, it is clear that the bone can be as much as fifty percent thinner than it was prior to the cast.

Because immobilization causes severe atrophy, or wasting away of the tissue, often when a person with OI comes out of a cast, he or she immediately refractures the bone. Then the cycle repeats itself. Many times, in mild cases of OI, the person may have had only ten fractures, but they have all been in exactly the same place. A terrible, vicious cycle of fractures can develop when bones become thin.

Summary

In summary, the pathology of OI is based upon an abnormality in collagen leading to inadequate connective tissue in general, and especially to impaired bone formation. The inadequate bone predisposes people to fracture easily. The fractures are responsible to a great extent for the deformities and for the growth deficiency. We probably will not find any sort of "magic bullet" in the near future that will eliminate the fractures, deformities, and other problems associated with OI. But there are things that we can do to help people with this disorder. The most important thing is to maximize physical development, because by maximizing muscular development we maximize bone development.

Works cited

Falvo, K.A., Bullough, P.G., *Osteogenesis Imperfecta: A Histometric Analysis, Journal of Bone and Joint Surgery, 55A:275-286, 1973.*

Falvo, K.A., Root, L., Bullough, P.G., *Osteogenesis Imperfecta: Clinical Evaluation and Management. Journal of Bone and Joint Surgery, 56A:783-793, 1974.*

Bullough, P.G., Davidson, D.D., Lorenzo, J.C., *The Morbid Anatomy of the Skeleton in Osteogenesis Imperfecta., Clinical Orthopaedics, 159:42-57, 1981.*

Endnotes

1. Sillence, D.O., Barlow, K.K., *Osteogenesis Imperfecta, A Handbook for Medical Practitioners and Health Professionals, Sydney, IMS Publishing, 1992, 7.*

2. Sillence, D.O., et al., *Osteogenesis Imperfecta Type II. Delineation of the phenotype with reference to genetic heterogeneity. American Journal of Medical Genetics 17:407-423, 1984.*

3. Thompson, E.M., et al, *Genetic Counselling in perinatally lethal and severe progressively deforming osteogenesis imperfecta. Annals of the New York Academy of Sciences. 543:142-56, 1988.*

4. Marini, Joan C., M.D., *Ph.D. Osteogenesis Imperfecta: Comprehensive Management, Advanced Pediatrics, 35:391-426, 1988, 400.*

5. Byers, Peter M.D., *personal interview, June 9, 1994.*

6. Sillence, D.O., Barlow, K.K. Ibid., 17.

Fig. 1-1	**Classification of Osteogenesis Imperfecta** [1, 5]		
OI Type	Clinical Features	Teeth	Inheritance
1A (IA)	Bone fragility varies from mild to severe; intensely blue sclerae; presenile hearing loss	Normal	Autosomal Dominant
1B (IB)	Bone fragility varies from mild to severe; intensely blue sclerae; presenile hearing loss	Opalescent Dentin	Autosomal Dominant
2 (II)	Extreme bone fragility, short crumpled bones, multiple rib fractures		New Dominant Mutation *
3 (III)	Variable but often severe bone fragility in infancy; progressive skeletal deformity; bluish sclerae	Variable dentin abnormality	Autosomal Dominant (usual) Autosomal Recessive (rare)
4A (IVA)	Bone fragility with normal sclerae; variable deformity	Normal	Autosomal Dominant
4B (IVB)	Bone fragility with normal sclerae; variable deformity	Opalescent dentin	Autosomal Dominant

* Recurrence in families generally is due to parental mosaicism for the altered gene.

Adapted from Sillence, D.O., Barlow, K.K., *Osteogenesis Imperfecta, A Handbook for Medical Practitioners and Health Professionals*, Sydney, IMS Publishing, 1992.

Figure 1-2 Radiographic Sub-Classification of OI Type II [2, 3]		
Subgroup	Radiographic Features	Recurrence Risk
A	Crumpled long-bones (accordion-like femurs), continuously beaded ribs due to numerous fractures	Less than 1%
B	Crumpled long-bones (accordion-like femurs), normal ribs or few fractures	6-7%
C	Long, thin fractured long-bones with thin wavy and beaded ribs	25%

Chapter 2

Prenatal Counseling and Diagnosis of Osteogenesis Imperfecta

by Melanie Pepin, MS and Peter H. Byers, MD
University of Washington

Introduction

In a given individual, if there is a family history of OI and physical features of OI are present, diagnosis can be very straight-forward. And on the other hand, when there is no history of OI in the family, and the physician is unfamiliar with OI, the correct diagnosis is not always obvious. Sometimes the circumstances surrounding the initial occurrence of fractures raise questions in the minds of observers, such as, "Could this be child abuse?" There are instances when specific diagnostic testing can establish or confirm the diagnosis of OI.

Diagnostic testing for any hereditary disorder comes in three forms:

- The direct detection of an alteration in a specific gene
- The demonstration that the "at risk" individual inherited the altered gene product from an affected parent
- The detection of the resulting protein abnormality

In OI, diagnostic testing most often involves study of the abnormal protein product, in this case, collagen. Gene screening or DNA testing is used less often.

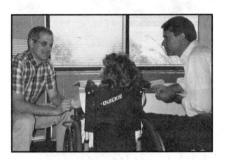

In every cell of the body we have two copies of two genes called COLIA1 and COLIA2. These two genes carry the information that directs a cell to synthesize a protein called collagen. Almost everyone who has OI has an alteration in one of the two copies of either COLIA1 or of COLIA2. There are twenty different types of collagen in our bodies that form the building blocks of bone, skin, and other tissues. The collagen type that is altered in OI is called type I collagen. Most people with OI each have a unique gene mutation and it is uncommon for two people with OI to have precisely the same genetic abnormality.

In some genetic disorders, the majority of affected individuals have an identical mutation that can be detected with relative ease. For example, almost all people with sickle cell disease have precisely the same change in the DNA of the B-globin gene that makes hemoglobin in red blood cells. In cystic fibrosis, about 70% of the altered gene copies have precisely the same change. For those disorders, developing methods to identify those very common changes makes sense. But in OI, where each person is likely to have a unique mutation, looking for a change in one of 18,000 COLIA1 or 38,000 COLIA2 building blocks of the collagen genes is currently time consuming and costly. The gene changes, even though subtle, may decrease the amount of collagen made, or they may change the structure of the collagen protein. Both these differences are relatively easy to detect and not costly to perform. Therefore, studying the collagen protein remains the most accessible and reliable diagnostic tool.

Does collagen testing identify all people with OI?

In the process of collagen testing we measure the amount of type I collagen that is manufactured by cells, and we determine whether the type I collagen has a normal structure. While these studies will identify the vast majority of people who have OI, approximately 15% of individuals with obvious features of OI do not demonstrate a collagen abnormality and therefore are not detected by this testing. There are two exact reasons for failure to identify all people with OI:

- In some people, the mutations are in other genes, although this is very rare.
- In other people, the genetic change produces protein changes that are too subtle to detect.

How is collagen testing done?

To examine collagen it is necessary to study cells that make type I collagen. Type I collagen is made in abundance by skin, bone, and other cells, but not by blood cells or by cells found in amniotic fluid. A small sample of skin, about 1/16 to 1/8 inch in width is taken from the individual suspected to have OI. This sample of skin is then minced and the very small pieces are covered with a liquid that encourages the skin cells to multiply. The cells are then incubated with a radioactive amino acid which is incorporated into the synthesized proteins. Those proteins are then harvested and examined. We do this by separating the proteins on gels which separate the proteins according to size. The larger proteins run more slowly and are thus above the small, faster migrating proteins in the gel. In the proteins from the person with OI, there are the two normal $\alpha 1(I)$ and $\alpha 2(I)$ bands and, in addition, a slower band that migrates above each. The slower bands are derived from the abnormal collagen molecules.

Next the DNA molecules from the nucleus of the cells are isolated and the region of the gene that contains the mutation (or alteration) can be sequenced. In the example shown in figure 2-1, the sequence of the gene is read from the bottom toward the top of the gel. By studying the DNA sequence pictured here, you will notice that the short lines correspond with the small letters above them. In the normal copy of the gene, the sequence from the bottom of the gel to the top reads ACTGGT-GCTGCC__G__GGCCC. This sequence encodes the protein sequence threonine-glycine-alanine-alanine-glycine-proline. In the sequence of the altered copy of the gene, the underlined G has been substituted by A which results in an arginine in place of the glycine. (Figure 2-1)

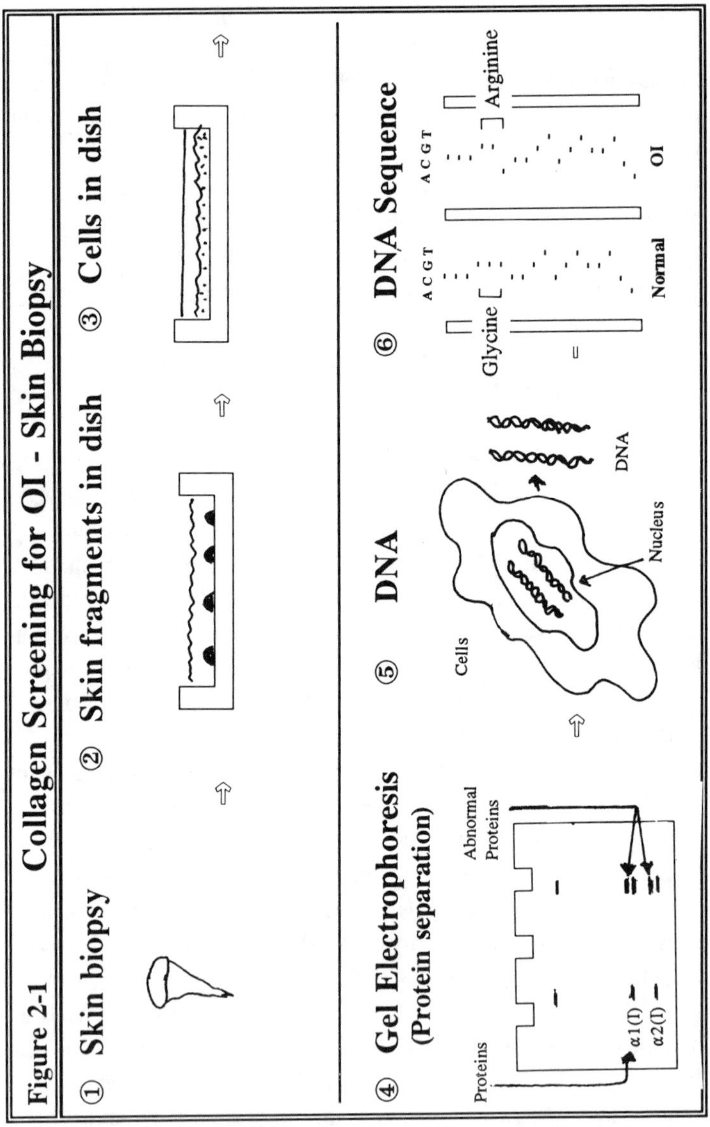

Figure 2-1   Collagen Screening for OI - Skin Biopsy

① Skin biopsy

② Skin fragments in dish

③ Cells in dish

④ Gel Electrophoresis
(Protein separation)

Proteins

Abnormal
Proteins

α1(I)
α2(I)

⑤ DNA

Cells

Nucleus

DNA

⑥ DNA Sequence

Glycine

A C G T   A C G T

Normal

Arginine

A C G T   A C G T

OI

About half a million cells are needed for the collagen studies. It may take four to six weeks to grow this many cells. These cells continue to make collagen even when they are outside the original tissue. When they are ready, we compare the amount and the structure of the type I collagen molecules and the products with molecules made by cells from a person who does not have OI.

Will collagen testing reveal the type of OI present?

For some individuals, we can tell whether or not the person has OI, and we can also determine the type of OI they have. We have learned that the cells from people with OI type I typically synthesize about half the normal amount of type I collagen. In other words, the amount made is abnormal. With this finding, now it is possible to determine, within a limited range, the severity of OI for that individual.

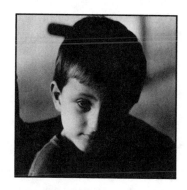

Cells from other people with OI, however, make a mixture of normal and abnormal type I collagen molecules. While the normal molecules perform their function as they should, the abnormal molecules stay in the cell for a longer time, and then, when, or if, they finally are sent outside, they interfere with the formation of strong bone. Many features of these altered molecules appear to determine the clinical effect; these include the type of thing wrong, the gene in which the mutation occurred, and where in the chain the alteration has occurred. At this point, there is too little information available on mutations and their clinical effect to allow an accurate prediction of given alterations. Furthermore, because similar effects on the proteins can result from quite different changes in the gene, we have to study many more people before we can determine how to predict the clinical outcome, given a certain change in the gene. Suffice it to say, at this point, the changes that permit a diagnosis of OI do not allow us to distinguish OI type II, or OI type III or OI type IV (with rare exceptions). Thus, because the "collagen screening" can be virtually identical in the different types of OI, we must rely on x-ray findings, clinical observation of the severity of the fractures and complications, as well as the degree of severity in affected relatives to predict the future clinical course for these individuals.

When should collagen testing be considered?

To decide whether to pursue collagen testing, the family, together with the physician, may want to examine whether collagen testing will answer the questions they have raised. Following are several circumstances in which collagen testing is often requested.

1. Testing for a child with mild OI

A child is suspected to have OI after his or her physician compiles findings from a physical exam, medical history, and family history. Collagen testing is useful to confirm the diagnosis of OI. This approach has it's limitations as the testing is not 100% accurate. We know that some affected individuals (about 10 - 15%), have normal collagen synthesis.

2. OI or child abuse?

Medical personnel are trained to pursue the possibility of "non-accidental trauma" or child abuse in cases of "unexplained fractures" or injury that appears to exceed the described trauma. An unfortunate set of circumstances can develop in situations where the child with OI is mildly affected with few diagnostic features beyond fractures. As you may guess, a physician may request a "child abuse" evaluation to exclude other signs of abuse. Physicians are required to report the incident to the state child protection services if abuse is suspected. False accusations of child abuse may have devastating emotional implications for families with a child with OI. Involving a medical specialist familiar with OI can often interrupt or limit such drastic measures. Collagen studies may be useful in this situation to confirm the diagnosis. It is important to remember that collagen testing is not 100% accurate so not all children with OI will be identified by testing. A collagen study indicating that OI is not detected, even though a 10 - 15% likelihood still remains that the results are in error, can work against a family in proving their innocence. In these cases, it may have been better for the child not to have been tested.

3. Testing an adult with OI

Collagen testing may be requested by an adult with OI. It may not be important to confirm OI by skin biopsy in adults who have a family history of OI in childhood. But if and when an adult with OI is planning a family, collagen testing will be most helpful in considering prenatal diagnosis.

4. Testing during pregnancy

Collagen testing may be requested for confirmation of the lethal form of OI (type II) detected in a fetus during pregnancy. With the advent of frequent ultrasound investigation in routine pregnancy care, more couples learn about OI when the presence of fractures, bowing, or under mineralized bones is identified during pregnancy. Infants with OI type II are often identified in this manner. The usual findings include shortened long bones, generalized under mineralization of bones, particularly the skull, bowing of the extremities and sometimes, fractures. There are a small number of other lethal genetic disorders that may be present in a similar fashion. If these abnormalities are identified early, some couples will opt for pregnancy termination, knowing the lethal nature of the disorder. Fetal cells from a skin sample or from the placenta can be studied for confirmation of OI. Identification of OI type II by ultrasound studies alone is probably quite accurate and may not need confirmation. Furthermore, the ultrasound findings are typically present by 14-16 weeks of pregnancy and skin biopsy studies would take an additional 3-4 weeks.

5. Genetic testing for families with OI

To understand how genetic testing for families with OI is possible, it is necessary to comprehend something about how people pass traits to their children through their genes.

The nucleus of every human cell contains 46 thread-like chromosomes. These 46 chromosomes come in 23 pairs, with one member of each pair coming from each parent. Genes, which are segments of DNA, are the basic units of hereditary information that reside on chromosomes and is passed from one generation to the next. There are two copies of every gene in every cell. Individuals with OI have an alteration in one of the two collagen genes, COLIA1, or COLIA2. Sperm in males and eggs in females contain only half of the 23 possible pairs, or half the number of possible genes. At conception the male and female cells unite to produce a new cell with 23 pairs of chromosomes - half from the mother and half from the father. It follows then that a person with OI will transmit an affected gene half the time and a normal gene half the time.

Occasionally, genetic testing for OI is available to large families with a number of affected individuals. Such testing may provide diagnosis in individuals, or during pregnancy, when the clinical findings are uncertain.

To offer this testing, we take advantage of normal variations in the gene sequences. These differences can be used in some families to determine which copy of the genes of Type I collagen (COLIA1 and COLIA2) contain the altered sequence that results in OI.

An example of how such studies might be used in a family is provided in figure 2-2. In this example, the grandfather (I-1) who has OI Type I, has two copies of the COLIA1 gene that we have called A and B, for convenience. The grandmother's copies are different and are called C and D. The four children of the grandparents, who we have called II-1, II-2, II-3, II-4, received different combinations of the genes from their parents as follows: II-1 has A and C; II-2 has B and C; II-3 has A and D; and II-4 has B and D. Of these, only II-1 and II-3 have OI. In the third generation, III-1 has A and D; III-2 has A and B, having inherited copy A of the COLIA1 gene from her unaffected and unrelated parent. III-1 has OI and III-2 is unaffected. Therefore, if the changed gene is a COLIA1 gene, the change that produces OI must be on the A copy of the gene. As you can see, in the next generation, only those people who received the A copy that came from the grandfather have OI. This is a simplified example of how this really works but shows how it is possible to determine which family members received the OI copy of the gene. (Figure 2-2)

Prenatal Diagnosis

Prenatal diagnosis of OI is available for some individuals and families. Diagnosis of OI during pregnancy can be accomplished by several means. The method of choice depends on the age at which bone deformity first becomes apparent, the family structure, the knowledge available concerning the nature of protein abnormality, and whether the precise genetic alteration is known. The diagnostic techniques include:

- Ultrasound evaluation of the fetal skeleton
- Chorionic Villus Sampling (CVS) - biochemical studies of collagen from cells grown from a biopsy of the placental tissue or genome testing to determine whether the OI gene copy has been transmitted to the fetus
- Amniocentesis for the sole purpose of fetal DNA collection

Ultrasound

Prenatal diagnosis by ultrasound is most useful to families at risk for the lethal and severe deforming varieties of OI which can be detected between 15 and 20 weeks of pregnancy. Fetuses with OI type IV can sometimes be identified, but often not until 24 weeks of gestation, if then. Rarely can infants with OI type I be identified through prenatally observing a fracture or bowing of long bones. And even then, these changes cannot be observed after 24 to 30 weeks of pregnancy.

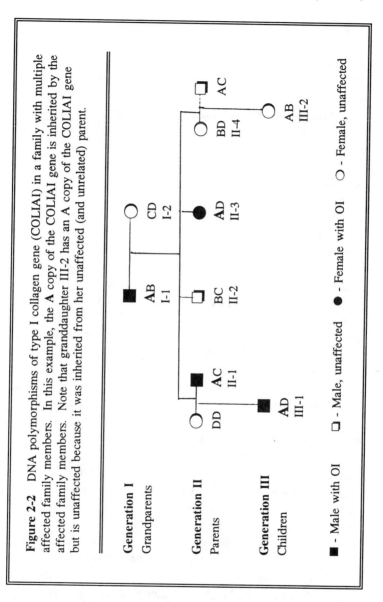

Figure 2-2 DNA polymorphisms of type I collagen gene (COLIAI) in a family with multiple affected family members. In this example, the A copy of the COLIAI gene is inherited by the affected family members. Note that granddaughter III-2 has an A copy of the COLIAI gene but is unaffected because it was inherited from her unaffected (and unrelated) parent.

Chorionic Villus Sampling (CVS)

Prenatal diagnosis can also be accomplished by a process called chorionic villus sampling (CVS). The tissue of the placenta originates from the fetus, and thus contains the same genes as the fetus. Experienced obstetricians who specialize in high risk pregnancies perform this procedure using special instruments and ultrasound. At approximately 10 weeks of gestation, CVS cells from the placenta are collected, and grown as described for a skin biopsy. Collagen studies are performed and these studies are compared with earlier studies performed on cells from the affected parent or previous affected pregnancy. Typically, results are available in about 3-4 weeks after the CVS procedure is performed. The prenatal collagen studies can only be offered if earlier collagen studies confirming the diagnosis in an affected relative have been completed.

Amniocentesis for the Sole Purpose of Fetal DNA Collection

In a family in which the precise genetic mutation has been identified or family DNA patterns studied, DNA can be extracted from CVS cells or from amniocytes collected by amniocentesis and studied to determine if the fetus has inherited the altered copy of the collagen gene. Amniocentesis, and studying the amniotic fluid, cannot be used to examine collagen synthesis as amniotic fluid does not contain a large enough quantity of cells that synthesize Type I collagen. The following chart will help explain the extent and the specifics of prenatal diagnosis for each type of OI. (Figure 2-3)

Summary

In conclusion, diagnostic testing of OI most often involves the study of type I collagen. Both the quantity of type I collagen manufactured by cells, and the quality of its structure is measured and compared with normal protein. For some, we can tell whether or not the person has OI, and we can also determine what type of OI they have. Collagen testing is often sought when testing for a child with features of mild OI, in attempting to diagnosis between OI or child abuse, and in testing for couples planning a family or during pregnancy. Genetic testing (or DNA testing) is available for multi-generational families with OI. Prenatal diagnosis of OI can be accomplished through ultrasound evaluation of the fetal skeleton, and in some cases by collagen screening performed on a sample derived from Chorionic Villus (CVS). Through continual investigation, and with the help of many people with OI, we hope to expand our knowledge of OI to provide improved genetic counseling for individuals, and to gain greater understanding of the molecular basis of this complex disorder.

Figure 2-3   Prenatal Diagnosis for OI

OI Type	Likelihood of Inheritance	Ultrasound	Collagen Screening by Analysis of Chorionic Villus Cells (CVS)	DNA Testing by CVS or Amniocentesis
OI Type I	• With one OI parent - 50% chance of recurrence	Not helpful since usually Type I OI births are fracture free. Could be performed late in the pregnancy.	Not reliable	Perform at 11 or 16 weeks. Much advance preparation involving many family members is necessary. Blood samples are studied.
OI Type II	• With one affected child: 5-6% likelihood • With 2 affected children, 20% likelihood	Perform at 14 - 17 weeks of gestation	Perform at 10 - 11 weeks. Earlier collagen studies of previous affected infant or pregnancy. Results take 3-4 weeks. Some risk involved	Perform at 11 or 16 weeks. Much advance preparation involving many family members is necessary. Blood samples are studied.
OI Type III and OI Type IV	• With 1 OI parent - 50% chance of occurrence • With one OI child - 4-6% chance of occurrence due to mosaicism	Perform first at 18 weeks gestation with follow-up ultrasounds at two week intervals. Interpretation depends upon the visible characteristics of the fetus	Perform at 10 - 11 weeks. Earlier collagen studies of affected parents are necessary and the results must provide an adequate basis for comparison. Results take 3-4 weeks. Some risk involved.	Perform at 11 or 16 weeks. Much advance preparation involving many family members is necessary. Blood samples are studied.

Chapter 3

Pregnancy and Osteogenesis Imperfecta

by Anthony Johnson, D.O.
Jeffersnon Medical College
Philadelphia, Pennsylvania

A woman with osteogenesis imperfecta (OI) who becomes pregnant can experience an uneventful pregnancy, or one laden with difficulties. Similarly, a developing fetus that is found to have OI can be born with very few complications, or it may not survive beyond a few hours. It is estimated that a woman with OI who becomes pregnant represents only 1 in 25,000 pregnancies that occur. Because OI is rare, and a pregnant woman with OI is even more rare, most obstetricians and other medical care providers will not have had experience in managing such cases.

Unfortunately, there is little data available at this time to allow us to speak with authority about the likelihood of a woman developing certain complications during pregnancy. In a recent review of the English medical literature, the author found only 18 reports involving 22 affected women who subsequently had 30 pregnancies. (Figures 3-1 to 3-4) The lack of consistency in reporting the various physical and laboratory findings, combined with the wide variance between people with OI, makes it quite difficult to draw any clear conclusions regarding a possible relationship between OI and many of the complications which have been reported thus far. Noting these limitations, this chapter will attempt to address some of the specific problems that have been suggested to be associated with OI. Also, management schemes will be proposed that may be beneficial in reducing the complications and negative affects of both the pregnancy of a woman with OI, and a baby born to either a mother with or without OI.

Obstetrical and gynecologic concerns of women with OI

A women affected with OI can expect to begin menstruating at the same time as an unaffected woman. Menstrual periods usually occur at the customary time, and cycles are generally regular. There may be heavy bleeding in women with a history of easy bruising or bleeding tendencies. While reproduction may be hampered due to the increased susceptibility to fractures or limited hip movement, there is no evidence to suggest that fertility or miscarriage rates are influenced by OI.

Pregnancy does not appear to have a significant adverse effect on the milder forms of the disorder. Women with OI types I and IV may experience loose joints, reduced mobility, increased bone pain and dental problems during pregnancy. In general, the medical concerns prior to pregnancy in these women will be limited.

Individuals with the more severe debilitating forms of OI who have short stature and curvature of the spine are at increased risk for both medical and obstetrical complications. If the level of curvature of the spine is great, the likelihood of heart and lung difficulties is increased. It is possible that these women will require early hospitalization due to increasing breathlessness. Premature delivery or even termination of a pregnancy may be necessary if signs of severe heart and lung problems develop, (cases 3, 12, and 19 in the chart that follows). As the pregnant uterus grows, the shortened distance from the thoracic cage to the pubic bone can cause discomfort and result in a need for extended bedrest.

Various obstetrical complications have been reported in women with OI, including preeclampsia, (characterized by hypertension, protein in the urine, and swelling), premature delivery, placenta previa (when the placenta becomes implanted in the uterus and covers the cervix), premature rupture of membranes, recurrent urinary tract infections, anemia, (low red blood cell count), and calcium deficiency. However, based on the available information it does not appear that there is an association between OI and these events. Another way to consider this concept is just because people with OI routinely catch a cold, we do not conclude that there is any association between OI and the common cold.

Pregnancy has not been associated with an increased risk of maternal fractures. However, trauma during pregnancy or minimal obstetrical manipulation at the time of vaginal delivery may result in fractures, (cases 14, 15, and 16). It has been suggested that because a risk does exist for a woman with OI to fracture during delivery and because there is potential for other complications, elective caesarean section should be the method of choice for delivery of most women with OI. Some of the reported complications during delivery include, the birth canal being too small to permit birth, uterine rupture, and hemorrhaging. A caesarean section would also be prudent if there is a history of previous pelvic fractures, contracted pelvis, or if the woman has a severe form of OI. However, in women with OI who have normal pelvic dimensions, there is no compelling reason not to undergo labor and vaginal delivery.

Bleeding disorders in OI are usually not a problem. In those cases reported to have excessive bleeding following delivery, each had some form of prior trauma during labor. Since blood coagulation and platelet parameters were normal in these cases, we suspect that the hemorrhage was due to the inability of the tissue to heal properly from the collagen defect found in OI. Women at greatest risk for bleeding would be those with a history of recurrent nosebleeds, easy bruising, or excessive bleeding following previous orthopedic procedures.

In the absence of clear indications of who may be at greatest risk for hyperthermia, (an increase in body temperature during anesthesia), spinal or epidural anesthesia would appear to be the safest approach. These anesthesia procedures, which involve the spine, may be difficult in some women with old vertebral compression fractures.

When either parent is affected with OI, the fetus is at risk of being born with OI as well. As shown in Figure 1-1, in the chapter titled, "OI - The Basics", the majority of individuals affected with OI have the autosomal dominant form. This would imply that there is a 50% chance in each pregnancy that the fetus will also have OI. Excluding OI, the risk of other congenital disorders resulting from pregnancies where one parent has OI is no greater than that of the general population.

Obstetrical consideration for unaffected women when OI is detected in the fetus

Sometimes, through ultrasound, OI is detected in the fetus of an unaffected mother. The ultrasound may have been ordered because of a previously affected pregnancy; however, the majority of cases are in women with no previous history of OI. In either situation, the diagnosis presents certain medical and ethical problems that must be addressed in order to direct the remainder of the prenatal care, including accuracy of the diagnosis, severity of the disorder, prognosis for survival and normal development, and mode of delivery.

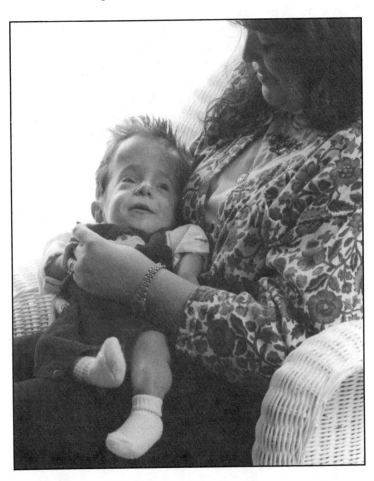

The age of the fetus when the ultrasound is performed, is important in order to achieve an accurate diagnosis and to provide the parents with the necessary information to consider all options for the remainder of the pregnancy. In pregnancies where OI type II is suspected, the studies performed prior to 24 weeks gestation should detect the severe shortening of the long bones and innumerable fractures in the limbs and thoracic cage. Fetuses with type III OI should also be detectable early in the second trimester due to the presence of multiple fractures and shortened limbs. When faced with this diagnosis, couples should be made aware that the former is uniformly lethal and the latter is often associated with significant disability and at times early mortality. It must also be stated that cases have been reported wherein the presumption that the infant would not survive has been discredited by children with severe forms of OI surviving and living very fulfilling and productive lives. While bowing of the long bones may be present in the second trimester, fractures in type I and IV may not be seen until the third trimester, if at all.

In regards to mode of delivery, it has been suggested that cesarean section would be less traumatic than vaginal delivery when fractures of the long bones of a fetus with types I, III, and IV OI are identified. However, women should be informed that there is no data to date which has shown this to be correct. Theoretically there is an increased risk of central nervous system injury with vaginal delivery when the baby's skull is poorly mineralized. Therefore it would be appropriate, when planning a mode of delivery, to assess the degree of mineralization in the baby's skull. Due to the grim prognosis in type II OI, the risk benefit ratio of elective cesarean should be discussed with the patient.

Ideally couples at risk due to parental and previous fetal OI should be seen for counseling prior to conception. Couples need to be made aware of the various complications which can be associated with OI and pregnancy. Discussion should include the availability of various prenatal diagnosis techniques including chorionic villus sampling, genetic amniocentesis, and second trimester antenatal ultrasound for the detection of OI. Otherwise there should be no need for deviation from routine prenatal care unless there is a reason why specialized care would be indicated. Weekly ultrasounds after 36 weeks gestation may be beneficial in detecting skeletal changes which may preclude vaginal delivery. Intrauterine pressure catheters and fetal scalp monitoring should be considered with vaginal deliveries due to the previous report of uterine rupture in labor.

While there are obviously increased maternal and fetal risks, women with OI should be made aware that the majority of women with OI who successfully conceive, withstand pregnancy quite well.

Table Codes: Figures 3-1, 3-2, 3-3, & 3-4,

Summary of Maternal and Neonatal Outcomes in 30 Pregnancies of Women with OI

Heading Codes

MA:	Maternal age
G:	Gravida (# of pregnancy this is for this woman)
P:	Paragravida (# of past pregnancies which resulted in a living baby)
GA:	Gestational age of the fetus (a baby is considered term at 38 weeks)
Mode:	Mode of delivery
Wght:	Birth-weight is measured in grams (to convert to lbs, divide weight in grams by 453.59)

Modes of Delivery and Complications of Pregnancy

SVD:	Spontaneous Vaginal Delivery
CS:	Cesarean Section
N/R:	Not Reported
PML:	Premature Labor
EAB:	Elective Abortion
CPD:	Cephalopelvic Disproportion (When the birth canal too small to permit vaginal birth)
SROM:	Spontaneous Rupture of Membrane
PFT:	Pulmonary Function Testing
ONTD:	Open Neural Tube Defect
HYS:	Hysterectomy
LF:	Low forceps
B-VE:	Breech birth with vaginal extraction

Figure 3-1   Summary of Maternal and Neonatal Outcomes in 30 Pregnancies of Women with OI

Author	Case #	Type OI	M A	G	P	Pregnancy Complications Before	During	After	Delivery Mode	Week	Neonatal Wght	Status
Greyman, JP 1962	1	I	19	1	0	none	none	none	SVD	Term	4040	blue sclera, no fractures
Plummer, D., 1982	2	I	27	1	0	x-ray 39 weeks, no fractures, thin bones	none	none	SVD	41	3680	blue sclera, fractured femur
Phillips, OP, 1991	3	III	21	1	0	ultrasounds, fetal skeletal deformities, of femurs, compromised maternal pulmonary status	N/R general anesthesia	N/R	CS	34	1685	type III OI
Carlson, JW, 1993	4	I	27	1	0	PML	none	none	EAB	37	N/R	Type I OI
				2	1	PML	N/R	N/R	SVD	8	3090	unaffected
				3	2	none	none	none	SVD	term .38	3000	unaffected
				4								
Young, BK, 1968	5	III	14	1	0	none	none	none	EAB	"20"	N/R	unaffected
	6	III	20	1	0	CPD	none	none	CS	41	2780	ONTD hydrocephalus, no OI
	7	I	25	1	0	pregnancy induced, hypertension, twins, CPD	none	post-op fever	CS	40	N/R	twins unaffected

Figure 3-3 Summary of Maternal and Neonatal Outcomes in 30 Pregnancies of Women with OI

| Author | Case # | Type OI | M A | G | P | Pregnancy Complications | | | Delivery | | | Neonatal | |
						Before	During	After	Mode	Week	Wght	Status
Johnson, WA, 1957	15	I	28	1	0	none	none	none	SVD	term	3290	blue sclera, no fractures
				2		none	laceration of vaginal mucosa & anal sphincter, 500 cc blood loss	severe tailbone pain, blood oozing at IV & injection sites	B-VE	42	3600	blue sclera, no fractures
Staples, PP, 1954	16	I	18	1	0	none	none	incomplete fracture of pelvis	LF	40	3147	blue sclera, no fractures
	17	I	23	1	0	pre-term delivery	N/R	N/R	N/R	N/R	1616	neonatal deaths, OI status N/R
				2	1	none	laceration of vagina, manual extraction of placenta, 1200 cc blood loss	none	LF	39	3147	blue sclera, no fractures
Graffeo, LW, 1953	18	I	32	1	0	none	none	none	SVD	N/R	2348	blue sclera, bowed thighs & legs
				2	1	N/R	N/R	N/R	SVD	N/R	N/R	unaffected

Figure 3-2   Summary of Maternal and Neonatal Outcomes in 30 Pregnancies of Women with OI

Author	Case #	Type OI	MA	G	P	Pregnancy Complications			Delivery			Neonatal
						Before	During	After	Mode	Week	Wght	Status
Young, BK, 1968	8	I	32	1	0	none	none	none	SVD	term	2360	unaffected
				2	1	32 week admission for massive edema & heroin withdrawal; 36 weeks, SROM	Excessive bleeding, uterine rupture	death 40 hrs after birth	SVD	36	2000	unaffected
Roberts, JM, 1974	9	I	21	N/R	N/R	recurrent urinary tract infections	none general anesthesia	none	CS	34	1660	unaffected
Key, TC, 1978	10	I	22	1	0	none	none	none	CS	39	3200	unaffected
Evans, HD, 1966	12	III	34	1	0	PFT vital capacity 975 ml, PML, 34 wks, CPD	none general anesthesia	none	CS	34	1660	unaffected
Bender, S., 1965	12	III	34	1	0	PFT: vital capacity 500 ml, comprised pulmonary function	none general anesthesia	none	HYS	16	N/R	ONTD
White, CA, 1963	13	I	23	1	0	none	none	none	SVD	42	3820	unaffected
Cohn, SL, 1962	14	I	23	1	0	38 wks SROM, slipped fractured pelvis & femur	none	hip-nailing, 3PPD, uneventful recovery	LF	38	N/R	unaffected

Figure 3-4   Summary of Maternal and Neonatal Outcomes in 30 Pregnancies of Women with OI

Author	Case #	Type OI	MA	G	P	Pregnancy Complications			Delivery		Neonatal	
						Before	During	After	Mode	Week	Wght	Status
Willard, WG, 1993	19	III	N/R	1	0	compromised maternal pulmonary status	chloroform anesthesia, difficulty breathing while side or back lying	none	HYS	"24"	N/R	N/R
Chernenak, FA, 1982	20	I	18	1	0	ultrasound 24 wks, bowed femur, 28 wks, femurs angulated femur,	none	N/R	CS	38	2900	osteoporosis blue sclera, fractured femur
Tsipouras, P, 1987	21	IV	31	1, 2	0, 0	SAB CVS at 8 wks, unaffected; PML 28 wks	N/R	N/R	CS	8, 34	2100	unaffected
Sengupata, B., 1987	22	III	28	1	0	excessive sweating, breathing difficulty while lying,28 wks, preeclampsia, CPD, x-ray bowing of fetal limbs & healing fractures, poor mineralization of skull	none	hemorrhage 72 hrs	CS	36	2380	fractured humerus, soft skull with wormian bones

Chapter 4

Healthy Eating for Children with OI

by Rosemary Parisi, R.D.
National Institutes of Health
Bethesda, Maryland

In general, children with osteogenesis imperfecta (OI) have the same nutritional needs as other growing children. Children with OI are sometimes different from other children in that they are often short statured, osteoporotic, and have decreased lean body mass. While there is no evidence that suggests that diet can prevent or cure this disorder, children with OI should eat a healthy diet to promote optimal health. This chapter provides information about the nutritional needs of children with OI and gives guidelines on how to provide a healthy diet. In addition, children with OI often develop truncal obesity, are constipated and perspire profusely. Suggestions for addressing these problems are also included.

Nutritional Needs of Children with OI

Most children who eat a variety of healthy foods will get the nutrients they need to grow. Essential nutrients include carbohydrates, protein, fat, vitamins, and minerals.

Carbohydrate:

Carbohydrate is the major source of energy for the body. The principal dietary carbohydrates are complex (starch), and simple (sugar). Starch is found in bread, cereal, pasta, and starchy vegetables such as potatoes, peas, corn, and lima beans. Sugar is found in two forms: natural which is found in fruit, fruit juices, honey, and refined, (white sugar) found in cookies, candy, and sweetened drinks.

Protein:

The primary function of protein is to build and maintain body tissues. Protein is found in meat, fish, poultry, eggs, milk and milk products, dried beans, peanut butter, nuts, and seeds. Most children get more than enough protein for growth.

Fat:

Fat is a ready source of energy. Primary sources of fat are butter, margarine, oils, mayonnaise, and salad dressings. Fat is also found in foods such as meats, dairy products (milk and cheese), desserts (pies, cakes, cookies), pastries, most snack foods, and many fast foods. Sometimes fats are used in food preparation methods such as frying or sauteing, in gravies, sauces, or added as seasonings. The intake of fat should be moderate.

Iron:

Iron is needed in the diet to prevent iron deficiency anemia. Children eating adequate amounts of meat, poultry, fish, enriched breads, cereals, and pasta (as outlined in Figure 4-3), are more likely to get an adequate amount of iron. A food rich in vitamin C consumed at the same time as an iron rich food will improve absorption of iron.

Vitamin A:

Vitamin A is an important vitamin in growth, vision, development and maintenance of skin and bone, and in fighting infection. To assure that a child is getting adequate Vitamin A, include at least one serving of a Vitamin A rich fruit or vegetable every other day. The best fruit sources for Vitamin A are: apricots, cantaloupes, mangos, papayas, nectarines, plums (canned), and prunes. The best vegetable sources of Vitamin A are: asparagus, broccoli, carrots, peas, spinach, sweet potato, cabbage, brussels sprouts, kale, collard greens, red sweet peppers, pumpkin, water squash, tomato, vegetable juice. Dairy products are also a good source of Vitamin A.

Vitamin C:

Vitamin C has many functions in the body. It is important for people with OI because one of its primary functions is to aid in the production of collagen. Collagen is necessary for the formation of connective tissue in tendon, bone, cartilage, skin, and tooth dentin. Collagen is also involved in the healing of fractures. Children should receive at least one Vitamin C rich fruit or vegetable each day. The best fruit sources are: orange, grapefruit, tangerine, and the juices of these fruits: nectarine, strawberries, mandarin oranges, kiwi fruit, cantaloupe, honeydew melon, papaya, mango, and any juice that has been fortified with Vitamin C. The best vegetable sources are: broccoli, tomato, tomato and vegetable juice, sweet potato, baked potato, green and red pepper, cabbage, brussels sprouts, kale, and Swiss chard.

Calcium:

Calcium is needed for adequate mineralization and maintenance of growing bones. To date there is no evidence that intake above the RDA (or 800 mg. per day for children age 1-10) will prevent osteoporosis. Osteogenesis imperfecta is a genetic disorder of the connective tissues, not a disorder of calcium intake or metabolism. Excessive amounts of calcium given as supplements may harm a child's kidneys. The best sources of calcium are milk and diary products, but other foods can also contribute. A child can get adequate amounts of calcium by drinking 2-3 cups of milk each day. If the child is not a milk drinker, a cup of yogurt or two ounces of cheese can be substituted for one cup of milk. To further encourage milk drinking, try limiting the amount of juice, fruit drinks, and soda. Also, if a child sees other family members drink milk regularly, the child will be likely to follow suit. Listed below are some ideas for increasing calcium intake in the diet:

• Offer fruit-flavored yogurt as a snack or topping on fruit.
• Use cheese in cooking. Melt it on sandwiches or vegetables. Grate and add to casseroles, soups, sauces, mashed potatoes, noodles, rice, meatloaf, or scrambled eggs.
• Use fortified milk: Combine two cups of fluid milk with 1/3 cup powdered milk. Refrigerate and substitute whenever you use milk in cooked cereals, soups, gravies, and puddings instead of water.
• Add powdered milk to casseroles, meatloaf, and sauces.
• Add flavorings to milk, like strawberry or chocolate, and make eggnog, cocoa, or milkshakes.
• Blend milk or yogurt with fruit to make a milkshake type beverage.
Some children may get stomach cramps, diarrhea, or intestinal gas after drinking milk. They may have an intolerance to lactose, the natural

sugar in milk. Try using low-lactose milk, which is available in most supermarkets, or ask your pharmacist for products that can be used to reduce the lactose in regular milk.

Vitamin and Mineral Supplements:

In current medical practice, vitamin-mineral supplements are not recommended unless there are special needs or intolerances to many foods. If a child consumes a variety of foods on a daily basis, he will most likely receive adequate amounts of vitamins and minerals for growth. Many parents, however, give their children vitamin-mineral supplements, in which case a pediatric multivitamin-mineral that provides up to 100% of the USRDA is recommended. Check with your doctor or dietitian before using any supplement. Excessive amounts of vitamins or minerals should be avoided.

Providing an Adequate Diet for a Child with OI

It is important that children with OI consume adequate amounts of nutritious foods for optimal growth and development without excessive weight. Children's appetites and intakes can vary from day to day, and sometimes decrease for long periods of time. Struggles over food can develop between parent and child during these times. Parents should remember that the quality and variety of food eaten is more important than the quantity.

Figure 4-1 is a guide for food and portion sizes to provide an adequate well balanced diet for children of different ages. Food for both meals and snacks can be selected from this guide. No single food group can supply all the nutrients needed. A nutritious diet must include a variety of foods.

Snacks: Most children eat four to six times per day, making snacks as important as meals in contributing to the total nutrient intake. Snacks should be carefully chosen. Any food that is appropriate for a meal is appropriate for a snack. (See **Figure 4-2** for a list of nutritious snacks.)

As a rule, limit snack foods such as chips, snack cakes, most cookies, sweetened fruit drinks, soda, and candy. These foods are high in calories and provide few, if any, nutrients. Snacks should be offered midway between meals. They should be offered long enough after the previous meal so that the child knows he will have to go hungry for some time if he refuses a meal. It is important for parents to remember that they have control over the timing of snacks and the type of snack food that is offered.

Weight Control

The medical consequences of being overweight for children with OI include stress on already brittle bones, and weak joints. Overweight can also place stress on the cardio-pulmonary system. Little is known about the actual caloric needs of children with OI. It appears that their caloric needs can vary depending on the severity of their disease and their level of physical activity. Generally, children with OI should be eating less than their peers. The best way to keep their calories at the right level is to limit high-calorie, low-nutrient foods, such as chips, cakes, cookies, candy, soda, and sweetened fruit drinks. Children with OI should be allowed to eat as many healthy foods as they want. Avoid attempts to withhold food, since this can set up struggles between parents and children. It is the parents' responsibility to provide nutritious meals and snacks at regular times and to control the eating environment. It is also important for parents to model good eating habits.

Strategies for Weight Control

1. Provide only nutritious foods and limit fat and sugar in the diet: Plan meals that contain a protein source, a carbohydrate source, and a small amount of fat. Use more starchy foods like bread, potatoes, noodles, cereal, and less foods that contain sugar. Be careful not to add fat or high-fat sauces to starchy foods. Use calorie-dense foods sparingly. Any food that is fried or has added fat is going to be high in calories. Many foods high in fat are also high in sugar. Try gradually reducing the amount of high-fat foods and high-sugar foods that you serve. Limit beverages to low-fat milk or skim milk (for children older than age two), unsweetened juice, and water. Offer low-fat yogurt and cheese. Use low-fat or skim milk in puddings, soups, and baked products. Substitute plain low-fat yogurt or blender-whipped, low-fat cottage cheese for sour cream or mayonnaise. Choose lean cuts of meat such as round, loin, sirloin, or lean hamburger and serve chicken, turkey, and fish more often. Trim all visible fat and remove skin from poultry. Choose cooking methods carefully; i.e. roast, bake, broil, or simmer meat, poultry, and fish. Steam, boil, or bake vegetables. Better yet, serve vegetables raw. Use non-stick vegetable sprays to reduce added fat when cooking and season vegetables with herbs and spices instead of fatty sauces, butter or margarine.

2. Control the eating environment: Set regular eating times for meals and snacks. Prepare low-calorie, low-fat foods for the whole family. Limit eating to one or two appropriate places in the home. Encourage children to eat slowly and enjoy the meal. Use small plates. Store food out of sight and out of reach. For example, keep cookies in an opaque container on a high shelf, or even better, do not have high-calorie and high-fat foods in the house at all. Prepare only enough food for one or two servings per person, or serve on plates directly from the stove, rather than from serving bowls on the table. Reassure a child that if he wants more, he can have more.

3. Encourage physical activity as your child's medical condition permits: Swimming is one of the safest exercises for children with OI. The kind and amount of physical activity should be determined individually in consultation with your child's doctor and/or physical therapist.

Constipation

Constipation is a problem frequently experienced by people with OI. It may be the result of limited physical activity, low fluid intake (particularly when there is excessive perspiration), a low-fiber diet, and/or medications. A high-fiber diet, adequate-fluid intake, and appropriate physical activity may relieve or prevent constipation. Introduce a variety of high-fiber foods to your child's diet gradually. Sometimes intestinal gas is a common problem with higher fiber diet, but it usually subsides within a few weeks.

The following tips may help to increase dietary fiber: Offer daily servings of fruits. Apples, oranges, blueberries, strawberries, peaches, pears, dried fruits, and prunes are good sources of fiber. Offer more raw and cooked vegetables daily. Broccoli, carrots, corn, green peas, potatoes with skin, green beans, peppers, brussel sprouts, radishes, and cucumbers are good sources of fiber. Offer more whole grain breads and cereals and whole grain flours, such as wheat, corn,oats, and their brans. Try brown rice, air-popped popcorn, whole wheat breads (choose bread that contains whole wheat flour), and whole wheat spaghetti. Replace half of the white flour in cake, cookies, and muffin recipes with whole grain flour. Serve high-fiber, ready-to-eat cereals. Add unprocessed bran or bran flakes to casseroles, meatloaf, soups, baked goods, muffins, and cookies. Encourage children to drink fluids – water is preferred for those who perspire.

Conclusion

In conclusion, this chapter has provided guidelines to parents of children with OI to help assure a healthy diet for optimal growth and development. It has also discussed some nutritional problems that children with OI may have. Parents who offer a variety of healthy foods with a casual, easy attitude about how much their child eats, can help a child with OI to build good eating habits.

For Figures 4-1 and 4-2, see Appendix F, pages 286 and 287.

Chapter 5

Rehabilitation, Physical Therapy, Orthotics and the Child with OI

Lynn H. Gerber, MD, Chief, Department of Rehabilitation, National Institutes of Health, Bethesda, MD
and
Joan C. Weintrob, CPO
Orthotic Prosthetic Center, Inc., Fairfax, Virginia

The rehabilitation of each child with osteogenesis imperfecta is determined by his or her unique needs and individual goals. The bone structure, muscle strength, developmental stage, motivation, and interests differ with each individual. Through a multi-disciplinary approach to the rehabilitation management of infants and children with OI, we have developed a program which focuses on increasing functional activity and helping the child become better integrated physically and socially into society. This approach, based upon a research protocol currently being conducted at the National Institutes of Health in Bethesda, Maryland, incorporates input from physical therapists, orthopedic surgeons, physiatrists, orthotists, and pediatricians. Together we provide a coordinated program with the following goals:

- Preventing abnormal postures
- Strengthening of the large muscles needed to support the body in the upright position
- Identifying developmental and cognitive deficits
- Devising strategies for bracing and surgery to support ambulation
- Educating the family, school personnel, and others about OI

We believe that through correct education, positioning and treatment designed to strengthen muscles, and improve stamina, even severely affected people with OI can experience increased independence and an improved quality of life. Also, if a conscientious rehabilitation program is followed through the formative years, many children are able to achieve levels of independence and mobility rarely seen in children of preceding decades.

Even though the degree of disability may be severe, management of children with OI should not be limited to just orthopedic procedures and bracing. Though ambulation, for some children, may not be a realistic goal, it is still important for the parents to help the child learn appropriate positioning to provide relief of discomfort and prevent deformities. The quality of life for children severely affected by OI can be improved considerably if measures are taken early on to encourage full function and interaction within society.

Positioning

How a child with OI lies or sits during infancy can affect their ultimate ability to sit, stand, and walk. Through the first years of life, parents should regularly turn a child from side to side when he/she is lying down. It greatly benefits the child to lie on the stomach if possible. Sometimes the prone position cannot be maintained because of respiratory problems, large head size, abnormal chest configuration, or fractures of the upper limbs. If this is the case, sandbags or towel rolls can be placed between the knees while side-lying. These positioning methods will help

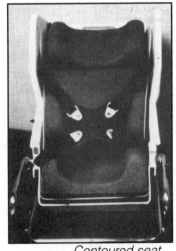

Contoured seat

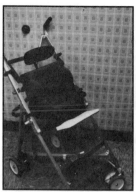

Contoured seat fitted into a stroller

prevent hip contractures, which, unless monitored, can become an obstacle to future sitting and standing.

Infants with OI are often delayed in their gross motor development and growth and hence their passage through important milestones is delayed. The more severely affected child often has a large head, weak neck and trunk muscle, and trunk control. Head and trunk control are essential for sitting and standing. If a child is unable to lift his/her head, or sit unsupported, a contoured seat, should be used. It is designed to fit into an infant seat, stroller, or wheelchair. Initially the seating system can be tilted but as the child gains more trunk control it can be brought to a more upright position. The seating system should have a head rest, seat belt, chest support and foot rest. It should attempt to prevent the legs from spreading into a frog-leg position.

We have found the optimal seating system to be one that is contoured to the child. The system we recommend for infants and very small children is multilayered and fits into an infant seat. As the child grows, layers of foam can be removed to accommodate for growth. This is definitely a more cost effective approach to the seating challenge. Another advantage of this seating system for children is that it provides head and trunk support.

A lap tray is provided to encourage the child to engage in daily living and play activities. As the child gains head control, the head rest can be removed. If possible, while sitting, the child should be positioned with the hips, knees, and ankles bent at 90 degrees. The knees should be close together. The child should sit with knees bent and feet supported to reduce stress on the back, which may potentiate compression fractures.

Physical Therapy

Exercises designed to promote head and trunk control are initially recommended. Also, exercises geared to improve stamina are needed for the child with OI. Swimming and water play are ideal for these children. To be of maximum benefit, therapy should begin as soon after birth as possible. The physical therapist works with the child in a developmental sequence starting with head and trunk control, moving next to sitting balance, propping and crawling, standing balance, and ending with ambulation, if feasible.

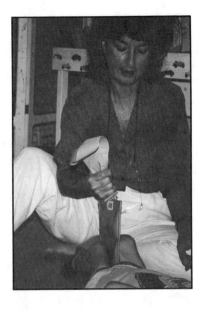

Anticipation of the future needs of the child by assessing motor development potential is very important, but at times difficult. Currently there is no sure method to determine the potential for physical achievement of a child with OI. However, it can generally be stated that a child with head control is usually able to achieve trunk control and the ability to sit independently. Independent sitting is necessary before one recommends standing.

Many children with poor joint alignment, poor balance, suboptimal gait patterns, and low endurance can be treated and may subsequently be able to stand and walk. At this point, we are not always able to predict who will advance to ambulation. Depending upon the individual child, a rehabilitation program could include:

- Posture exercises - sitting and standing when appropriate
- Active range of motion exercises - especially for hip girdle muscles and to stretch hip flexors
- Therapeutic and recreational water activities
- Standing
- Strengthening exercises
- Stretching
- Cycling - "Hot Wheels," etc.
- Prone progression
- Transfers - from floor to chair, chair to bed, etc.
- Ambulation
- Coordination exercises

Parents should seek the council of experienced medical professionals who will design a program of physical therapy and overall rehabilitation individualized for their child.

Considerations for Bracing and Standing

The readiness of the child for upright activity should be determined as the child gains head and some trunk control. The decision to begin standing is based on many factors. These include:

- Developmental stage - head and trunk control
- General muscle strength
- The laxity or tautness of the joints
- The fragility of the ribs
- The nature of the bony structure of the long bones
- The degree of bone curvature, including scoliosis
- The history of fractures
- The level of motivation of both the child and family

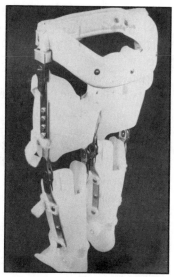

Children with OI often have very flexible, lax joints. The knees can go into a backward posture, the feet appear flat, and the trunk is bent over the legs. These mechanical problems often progress throughout life. Children who are weak and have ligamentary instability are likely to benefit most from bracing. The bracing consists of a long leg, clamshell-type orthosis with knee and hip joints and a pelvic (hip)

Clamshell type braces

band attachment. The knee and hip joints allow for comfortable sitting and normal reciprocal ambulation.

The incidence of scoliosis is extremely high in children with OI. Spinal bracing is usually poorly tolerated and has not been shown to be effective in controlling scoliosis. The corrective force exerted by a back brace on the bones of children with OI can do more harm than good. Bracing for scoliosis can cause progressive rib deformity rather than correct a spinal deformity. Treatment for scoliosis usually requires surgical intervention.

If the bones of the lower extremities are significantly curved, or children have had multiple fractures of long bones of the legs over a relatively short period of time, orthopedic surgery should be considered. The role of orthopedics becomes critical when deciding to brace a child with OI. If standing and walking is the goal, it may be necessary to undergo a surgical procedure designed to straighten a curved bone, or support a curved bone with a rigid internal device.

In our program at the NIH, the youngest child we have recommended for bracing was eight months of age, but most are between two and five years of age. If a child has not walked by age five, he or she is unlikely to walk without rehabilitation intervention, possibly with orthopedic or orthotic assistance.

Our experience with children with OI has shown that bracing appears to have no influence on femoral bowing, but tibial bowing may be slightly decreased. The beneficial aspects of bracing is improved joint alignment in the hips, knees, and ankles foot complex. Some children gain the ability to walk earlier than they would have without braces and children walking with braces have a more normal, steady gait pattern. Children in braces tend to be more active than those who do not wear them, and these children engage in more varied and strenuous physical activities.

Bracing Information for the Child with OI

When bracing a child with OI, it is extremely important that the orthotist take accurate preliminary measurements. These measurements become the blue print for fabricating a well-designed brace. A plaster mold is taken of each leg as well as linear and circumferencial measurements of the legs and hip region. During the molding process it is very important to achieve optimum alignment of the legs. The orthotist is always extremely careful in removing the cast to avoid causing a fracture.

There are many types of braces available. The type that is needed for a specific child is determined by the amount of muscle strength and/or joint alignment. Some of the bracing options for children with OI include:

HKAFOs - Hip Knee Ankle Foot Orthoses

These are for children with pelvic girdle instability and general lower extremity weakness. Some children also require rotational control at the hips.

KAFO - Knee Ankle Foot Orthosis

This type of brace may be used to control valgus or varus deformities of the knee, support weak muscles of the legs, or provide support for a healing fracture.

AFO - Ankle Foot Orthosis

This type of brace may be used to support weak muscles of the lower leg and foot, control severe deformities and joint laxities of the foot, or provide support for a healing fracture.

SMO - Supramalleolar Orthosis

This type of brace is used primarily to control deformities of the foot, such as hindfoot valgus or flat feet.

The perfect fit

It is important that braces fit comfortably and are easy to wear. Lighter weight knee and hip joints and thermoplastics are most appropriate for people with OI. To accommodate the heat intolerance experienced by many people with OI, we generally drill holes through the plastic of the front calf and thigh sections of the orthoses which allows for maximum air circulation.

Photo by Laura Vinchesi

Standing Frame

The braces are initially used along with a simple standing frame. The child, in his or her braces, can be strapped into this frame and allowed to bear weight while unattended.

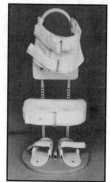

Standing frame

Walking

Once orthopedic and rehabilitation specialists agree that the child is safe for ambulation, a program to help the child learn to walk can begin. Even though some may not progress beyond indoor ambulation, the ability to walk will make them much more independent and may result in increased bone mineralization. The ambulation program we recommend begins by walking with the aid of braces or parallel bars, then with a pushcart or walker, progressing to crutches, a cane, and

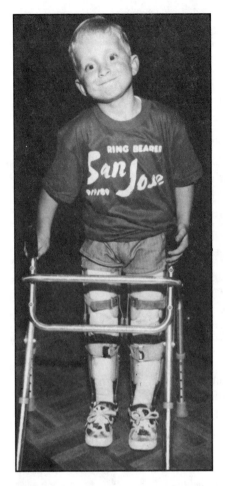

with good fortune, eventually the child may be able to walk unassisted. It is important to know that every child with OI does not need braces to be able to walk. Some children walk independently without the aid of braces. It is also possible that a child, who walks without the aid of braces, could have walked earlier with braces. The benefits of bracing and the risks of bracing for children with OI are currently being studied at the National Institutes of Health.

Fractures Can Limit the Rehabilitation Program

Children in casts undergo many changes as a result of the trauma. They often regress socially or are more socially isolated. They are less mobile and refrain from using the casted limb, resulting in bone demineralization and muscle weakness. Endurance and stamina also decrease.

The post-fracture period is a very critical one. The reintroduction of standing, walking, and strengthening must be undertaken very cautiously to prevent the bone from refracturing. A review of the femur fracture incidence of 32 children with OI, showed the greatest danger period for refracture to be the first six months. Two-thirds of recurrent fractures occurred in this time period. Therefore, we conclude that physical therapy and hydrotherapy, possibly supplemented by bracing, should be temporarily increased after removal of the cast. Children are often wary of walking after a fracture, and need additional support and encouragement if they are to become confident of their abilities.

Conclusion

Most children with OI benefit from a rehabilitation program aimed at promoting functional independence. Walking is one aspect of this. Children with ambulation potential may benefit from bracing. If combined with strengthening exercises and preceded by surgical straightening procedures as necessary, many children with OI can become successful home or community ambulators.

Some children who are braced as toddlers may no longer need braces as they grow. The decision to wean from, or stop bracing, is not an easy one and few specific guidelines are available to help decide on a rational basis. Studies are underway at this time to help answer questions about whether and when to discontinue bracing.

In conclusion, a major effort is needed by persons from many disciplines, in conjunction with children, families, and school, if we are to safely and effectively rehabilitate children with OI. Using such an approach, many will be successfully integrated into the mainstream of society and reach a high degree of function.

Acknowledgement:

The team that has helped develop and execute this program include:

Physical Therapists:	Ann Conway, RPT, Roger Berry, RPT, and Joe Shrader, RPT
Orthotist:	Joan Weintrob, CPO
Physicians:	Lynn Gerber, MD, Helga Binder, MD and Joan Marini, MD
Orthopedists:	Michael Reing, MD
Registered Nurse:	Stephanie Bordenick, RN
Biochemist:	Karen Siegel, RPT, MS

Works Cited

Binder, H., Conway, S.H., Gerber, L.H., Marini, J., Berry, R., Weintrob, J., *Comprehensive Rehabilitation of the Child with Osteogenesis Imperfecta, American Journal of Medical Genetics,* 45:265-269, 1993.

Binder, J., Conway, A., Gerber, L.H., *Rehabilitation Approaches to Children with Osteogenesis Imperfecta: A Ten-Year Experience, Archives of Physical Medicine and Rehabilitation, Vol.* 74, 386-390, 1993.

Gerber, L.H., *Rehabilitation for Children with Osteogenesis Imperfecta, Breakthrough, The Newsletter of the Osteogenesis Imperfecta Foundation, Winter 1990.*

Weintrob, J., *Orthotic Management for Children with Osteogenesis Imperfecta, Address delivered at the Medical Frontiers Symposium, National Institutes of Health, 1992.*

Chapter 6

Dentinogenesis Imperfecta and other Dental Concerns

by Ronald J. Jorgenson, D.D.S., Ph.D.
South Texas Genetics Center, San Antonio, Texas

The problem

The dental problems experienced by people who have osteo-genesis imperfecta are often referred to as dentinogenesis imperfecta (DI), "opalescent dentin", "brown teeth" or "defective teeth". The name doesn't matter as long as a term is used that accurately describes the condition. It is also possible to have DI without having OI.

Teeth are hard tissues, just like bone. The cells that form the dentin of teeth are similar to those that produce bone. It has been found that approximately 50% of people with OI have defective teeth. When the first baby teeth erupt, at about six months of age, parents will be able to determine whether the child has dental problems. If the first teeth to erupt are white, the rest of the teeth will be white, and there is no need to be concerned about special dental care. If, on the other hand, the first teeth are blue or brown, the other baby teeth as well as the permanent teeth will be affected. There is wide variation in dental fractures in the permanent teeth. Some people with OI have teeth that are very mildly affected while others are severely affected and require considerable dental care.

Clinical manifestations

The manifestations of dental problems in OI include teeth that are brown and that wear excessively. Also the enamel fractures away from the tooth surface. The teeth are sometimes misshapen, with an excessive constriction at the junction of the crowns and roots of the tooth. The pulp chambers are not as well formed as they should be; they're obliterated by dentin. The roots are foreshortened and tapered.

The problem with the teeth in OI is an inherent weakness in the way the enamel is attached to the dentin. The enamel is perfectly strong, it's perfectly thick, and it's perfectly well colored. The problem is that the enamel does not grasp onto the dentin in the normal way. The dentin is inherently defective and also has a defective scalloping where it joins with the enamel. The reason the enamel breaks away is that it does not have a sufficiently

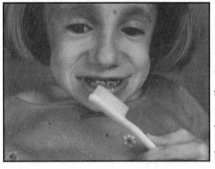

Photo by Smilen Savov

rough surface on which to grasp. The teeth appear brown in a person with defective dentition because there are spaces between the enamel and the dentin that allow the color of the dentin to show through.

Like the bony manifestations, the dental problem in OI tends to get better as time goes on. The most severely affected teeth will be those that develop the earliest. The least severely affected generally will be the ones that develop the latest. So, the front baby teeth ought to be the most severe, the back baby teeth less severe, the front permanent teeth less severe, and the back permanent teeth least severe of all.

Heredity

There does not seem to be a relationship between the severity of fractures in a person with OI and the degree to which the teeth are affected. It is important to know that the defect, when it exists in a family, breeds true in that family. In other words, when somebody in the family has OI and the brown teeth, everybody in the family with OI will have brown teeth. If somebody with OI has white teeth in a given family, everybody with OI in that family will have white teeth. This statement is made on the basis of experience with over 150 different families with OI. This information is helpful in diagnosing children born into families with a history of OI and opalescent teeth. If there has not been a firm diagnosis of OI prior to the eruption of the infant's first teeth, simply looking at the teeth can aid in that diagnosis.

Treatment

There is no way to prevent the problems associated with teeth in people with OI, just as fractures cannot be prevented. Nonetheless, it is important for people with OI to be earnest about proper tooth brushing and not to think that dental care is futile since the teeth will break and be lost anyway. We should remember that teeth are needed for a lifetime of chewing food properly, and tooth wear may result in abscesses and pain. Also, one of the primary purposes for baby teeth is to maintain proper spacing for the permanent teeth to erupt. If the baby teeth have been lost and are not present to act as placement guides for the permanent teeth, a bad bite could develop, requiring expensive orthodontic treatment later.

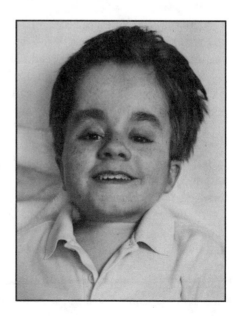

It would be rare to find a dentist who has treated more than one or two people with OI. Some may be reluctant to treat people with OI,

fearing jaw fractures. In truth, the everyday forces of chewing exert considerably more force on the jaw bone than does normal dental treatment. Fortunately, there have been no reports of people with OI experiencing jaw fractures as a result of standard dental treatment. It is important for children with OI to see a dentist as soon as the first tooth erupts.

Since we know that there is a deficiency in the interface of enamel and dentin, it is preferable not to leave the enamel and dentin undermined, as can happen when a dental filling is placed. Let's say somebody with OI has a cavity. The dentist might decide to treat the cavity fairly conservatively by removing the decayed area and putting in a filling. Unfortunately, while the dentist is making his cavity preparation the enamel may be undermined so that any force on the area around the filling is going to cause crumbling. Eventually that filling will be lost. It is very common for restorations to crack at the point where the biting force is applied. This happens quickly in people with OI who have the dental manifestation because of the inherent weakness. In this case, more aggressive dental treatment is recommended. Instead of a small filling, the dentist should consider a larger filling, or the use of a crown. In OI, the core of the tooth, or the root, is generally in good condition so it should be possible to maintain a crown for the life of the individual, as long as there are no exposed, weak surfaces that can crumble away.

One method of treating people who have dental problems of OI is to crown the teeth as they erupt. With baby teeth, it becomes difficult because the baby teeth are so small and children are sometimes unco-operative. The dentist, however, might consider crowning some baby teeth to maintain them for the time being. The back teeth are especially important since they help guide the permanent teeth into place, and are used for proper chewing throughout life. If the back teeth are too fragile or delicate as they erupt, they probably should be capped as quickly as possible. The teeth may be capped with stainless steel crowns. Porcelain crowns and gold crowns are more expensive, but may be a better treatment, especially for the permanent teeth.

Another method of treatment would be to extract whatever teeth are excessively broken down, then save and put permanent crowns over the rest. The objective is to save the roots. When roots are lost, the bone of the lower jaw is not properly stimulated and may resorb. When bone is gone, it becomes difficult or impossible to maintain a denture if necessary. Dentures, by the way, are perfectly acceptable forms of treatment for people with OI; that is, the bone is generally strong enough to tolerate the pressures caused by biting and chewing.

It is possible to use dental implants in people with OI. To insert a post, the dentist drills a hole, puts in a post, and lets the bone heal around it. Sometimes people with OI have jaw bones that may not be very thick or strong, which may not be able to accommodate implants. But if there is enough jaw bone and the jaws are properly aligned, it is better to use an implant than a denture.

A word of caution is in order about the use of bonding and composite resins. There is an inherent weakness in the bond between the enamel and the dentin in people with OI. This weakness can lead to the failure of restorations that do not cover the entire enamel surface. Whenever the restoration and enamel meet, then, there is bound to be a further loss of enamel. Even if the entire surface of the enamel were covered by some sort of composite, it is possible that the restoration may not be strong enough to withstand the forces of chewing.

Orthodontics

Orthodontics is sometimes considered for people with OI. Orthodontics involves moving a tooth through bone. When the tooth is pulled through the bone, resorption occurs on one side and healing on the other side as the tooth moves through. If there's a healing defect in

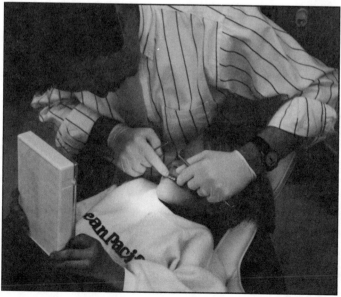

Photo by Chuck Glauser

OI, problems with orthodontics could arise because the jawbone may not heal properly if the tooth is moved extensively.

Fortunately, most people who need orthodontics don't need extensive movement of the teeth through the bone. All that is needed is a turning or a tilting of a tooth which is generally fairly successful in OI. Palette spreaders have been used successfully in people with OI. Extensive movement in people with very severe types of OI may present more of a problem. In milder types of OI, orthodontics should not present problems at all.

Cavities

One question that often arises is whether children with OI are susceptible to cavities since the enamel wears away from the dentin. They are not more susceptible to cavities. However, as the dentin is destroyed by cavities, the overlying enamel flakes away. So the enamel keeps pace with the dentin deterioration and the tooth wears away before it has a chance to get cavities. It is also true that missing teeth are as common in the general population as they are in people with OI.

Pain

People with OI do not necessarily have more dental pain than average. They may even have less pain because when the dentition is affected there is no pulp. The nerves of the teeth are in the pulp. A person with no nerves should not have pain. Generally speaking, dental pain is not a feature of OI.

Summary

Approximately 50% of people with OI have defective teeth. The problem, which manifests itself at the time of the first eruption of the baby teeth, is evident by worn, brownish teeth, where the enamel has fractured away from the tooth surface. There is no relationship between the severity of fractures in a person with OI and the degree to which the teeth are affected. Although, the defect, when it exists in a family, breeds true in that family, or when a family member has OI and the brown teeth, everyone in the family with OI will have brown teeth.

One method of treating people who have dental problems of OI is to crown the teeth as they erupt. Another method would be to sacrifice some teeth and put permanent crowns over the rest with the objective being to save the roots. Also, dental implants are used in the treatment of people with OI.

Chapter 7

Hearing Impairment in Osteogenesis Imperfecta

by Cheryl R. Greenberg, MD, CM, FRCPC, FCCMG
Winnipeg, Canada

Hearing impairment is often overlooked in the medical management of the person with OI, yet significant hearing loss is reported to be present in more than 50 percent of individuals affected with OI and often represents the most serious handicap. Prior to the average age of hearing loss in OI, (around 20 - 30 years), primary medical attention is usually focused on the treatment and care of fractures, overshadowing the development of hearing loss. However, symptoms may indeed be present earlier and are often not recognized. The nature and degree of hearing loss varies greatly with each affected person and within families, similar to the variability seen with other OI symptoms. To understand the nature of hearing loss in OI, it is important to review the normal anatomy of the ear and how it functions.

The Anatomy of the Ear

The ear is divided into three portions; the external, middle, and inner ear. The external ear includes the outer ear and the ear canal. Behind the ear drum at the end of the external ear canal, there is a small chamber called the middle ear. The three tiny bones, the malleus, incus, and stapes, which connect the ear drum and the inner ear, act in series to effectively transmit airborne sound through the middle ear to the fluid in the inner ear.

The important sensory organ of the ear is housed in a fluid filled area called the scala media. (See Figure 7-1.) When the vibrations of the small bones in the middle ear create waves in the inner ear fluid, the membrane, in which the sensory organ lies, is set in motion. This motion causes bending of the hairs of the sensory cells which transforms the mechanical energy to electrical energy and stimulates the auditory nerves. The information is then transmitted via the auditory nerve to the brain where the sound is interpreted and memorized.

A person who is hearing-impaired could have a problem in the middle ear, the inner ear, the auditory nerve, the brain, or in more than one of these areas.

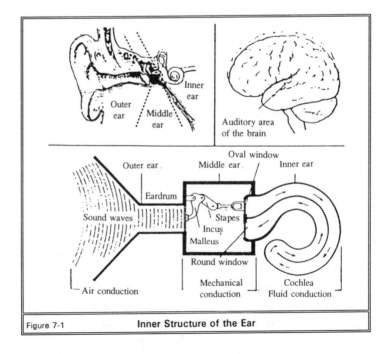

Figure 7-1   **Inner Structure of the Ear**

Types of Hearing Loss

There are three main types of hearing impairment:

- conductive hearing loss
- sensorineural hearing loss
- mixed hearing loss

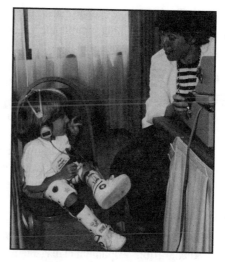

When hearing loss is caused by a physical problem in the external ear or in the middle ear, it is called a conductive hearing loss. When sound is conducted normally from the exterior ear though the tympanic membrane to the inner ear but when the inner ear, is not functioning in transmitting sounds normally to the brain, a sensorineural hearing loss is present. When both the middle and inner ear are involved, the hearing loss is called a mixed hearing loss. Hearing losses are also classified according to degree of severity: mild, moderate, severe, or profound, and according to whether or not the hearing loss affects low, high, or all the frequencies of sound.

Hearing Impairment in OI

The hearing impairment associated with OI can be either a sensorineural hearing loss, a conductive loss, or a mixed type. A large study conducted in Denmark by Pederson showed that 40 percent of people with OI have a conductive or mixed loss and 10 percent had a sensorineural loss. Another study conducted at the National Institutes of Health by Shapiro, Pikus, Weins, and Rowe suggested that sensorineural hearing loss occurred more commonly than conductive or mixed. Although in many individuals the hearing loss is mild, in others it can be moderate, severe, or even profound.

Why are people with OI prone to hearing loss? The otologic picture in OI has been compared to that seen in a more frequently encountered condition called otosclerosis. Although similar in some respects, the middle ear involvement is indeed different and usually more severe in OI. The footplate of the stapes becomes fixed and rigid and no longer transmits sound effectively to the inner ear. The generalized connective tissue defect seen in OI is also clearly manifested in the middle and inner ear with the bones of the tympanic ring, the middle ear, the cochlea, and the otic capsule being having a recognizable collagen defect. In particular, the stapes footplate undergoes significant change, becomes "fixed" or "floating." Some investigators have also reported that with increasing age, individuals with predominantly conductive hearing losses are found to have an increasing sensorineural component to the hearing loss. The cause of the sensorineural loss probably results from a variety of factors, including microfractures, bleeding, and overgrowth of fibrous tissue. This only compounds the degree of hearing impairment and increases communication difficulties.

Management of Hearing Impairment in OI

- **Recognition** – Optimum management firstly demands recognition of the problem. Thus, any child with OI who demonstrates a speech delay, recurrent ear infections, or articulation problems should have a formal audiologic assessment. Any adult with OI who complains of hearing loss and/or tinnitus (ringing in the ears), should undergo audiologic examination.
- **Amplification** – Appropriate hearing aids can be fit to a child or adult with a conductive, sensorineural, or mixed hearing loss. Very often hearing aids provide adequate amplification for effective and satisfying communication.
- **Surgery** – For the type of hearing loss called conductive, there is a surgical procedure known as a stapedectomy that has given very satisfactory results. Stapedectomy can be considered when there is a moderate to severe conductive loss. In this type of surgery, the fixed foot process of the stapes is viewed by the surgeon under a microscope through the exterior ear canal. The rigid stapes footplate is replaced by a Teflon prosthesis, which is secured into the oval window. This prosthesis would then allow for the normal propagation of sound waves to the inner ear.

  Although a stapedectomy is considered in many centers to be a commonly performed procedure for otosclerosis, this surgery should not be considered routine in people with OI. Because of tissue fragility seen in people with OI, great care must be taken to avoid fracturing the fragile stapes during the procedure. There are many other pre-operative and post-operative issues that need to be assessed, discussed, and clarified before any individual with OI may be considered a "good candidate" for surgery. Referral to a treatment center where physicians with considerable experience with OI are available is most important.

My Personal Experience

Many years ago as an undergraduate at McGill University, I learned the name of the disorder being transmitted in my family was Type I osteogenesis imperfecta. To make a long story short, I have been blessed to have a mild form of OI as have most members of my extended family including one of my two children. However, shortly after I gave birth to my first child, Matthew, I became aware that my hearing was significantly reduced. The audiologic assessment confirmed my suspicions - a mild to moderate conductive hearing loss in both ears. Amplification was prescribed, and I used my hearing aids with excellent results for a period of time. The hearing loss progressed in both ears to a moderate to severe conductive hearing loss. Somewhat apprehensively, I began to consider a stapedectomy.

Then one glorious summer day on a sandy beach approximately 60 miles north of Winnipeg, I lost my hearing aids in the sand. A tremendous sense of panic overtook me. Fortunately, I found the aids but from that day on I knew I was going to try the surgery. My 'Ear Nose and Throat' consultant, although experienced in stapedectomies, had limited experience with patients with OI, and was reluctant to "manually" mobilize the stapes footplate as is done in a routine stapedectomy.

I was referred to Dr. Coyle Shea in Memphis, and on March 9, 1987, underwent a stapedectomy on my left ear. Dr. Shea at that time used an argon laser to "zap" the foot process of the stapes and then insert a Teflon prosthesis. Following surgery I had essentially no problems with dizziness or pain, and my hearing improved dramatically to the point where I no longer wore my hearing aids. I am pleased to say that on July 9, 1991, Dr, Shea performed a stapedectomy on my right ear at the Memphis Surgical Center, this time using a specially designed steel micro-drill. Forty-eight hours afterwards, I was visiting Graceland, having had little if any post-operative discomfort. My hearing is now considered "normal" in both ears! Naturally, I hope this improvement is sustained long-term.

I would encourage anyone with a suspicion of hearing loss to first seek an audiologic assessment to learn if a hearing aid would be helpful, and then inquire if operative intervention is a realistic option. I realize that coming to terms with the reality of "hearing impairment" is difficult. It is just another piece in the whole puzzle of OI. There is too much to be lost if hearing loss is "ignored."

Tips for Effective Communication with A Person with a Hearing Impairment

1. Agree with me on a signal that can be used when: my voice is too loud; I'm monopolizing the conversation; my response is totally irrelevant because I heard wrong,(clue me in as unobtrusively as you can, or simply repeat some key words of what was said); I've interrupted because I failed to notice the speaker hadn't finished. If you can't catch my eye with your signals, try to tap me on the shoulder.

2. Keep hands away from mouth while you're talking. Also avoid scarves, cigarettes, and gum. Either trim your mustache or raise your voice.

3. Face me when you talk to me. Otherwise I need to keep moving, following you to get the whole message. If you need to leave the room, wait until we're together again to continue.

4. Don't shout. It distorts the words. My hearing aid does the amplifying. But don't drop your voice as you reach the end of a sentence.

5. Most people speed up their speech when they get excited or are in a hurry. It embarrasses me to ask you to slow down, so if I do it once, try to remember as you continue talking.

6. Don't exaggerate you enunciation. It makes you look different, and you are harder to understand. Sometimes you look funny, and I try not to laugh.

7. Don't call out from another room "I'm here." I may rush to get to you on the porch, when you're calling from the bedroom. Say "I'm in the bedroom."

8. If I've gotten a whole sentence wrong, repeat some of the words. The message that travels from my inner ear will reach my brain in time for me to catch up while you keep talking. It may even be better if you use a few different words to say the same thing, because the sounds you use the second time may be in a range that I can hear more easily.

9. You may expect me to hear as well on our porch as in the living room. But I usually hear better where there are soft drapes and carpets — anything that absorbs the peripheral sounds.

10. If you're having a lot of trouble communicating with me, I

may have had a hard day and feel tired, or I may be coming down with a cold or have a pain. Please make allowances.

Source Unknown

Ten Commandments for People Who Live with a Person who is Hearing Impaired

1. Be patient. Remember that a person who is beginning to suffer hearing loss is like a child beginning to talk, to listen, and to understand. All the conditions of communication are changing.

2. Accept reality, it changes both of your lives and introduces new elements in your relationship. It isn't going to go away.

3. Speak slowly. Consider what it's like for you when you listen to a newscaster on television who rushes through lines, especially when statistics are being quoted.

4. Don't shout. It doesn't help, and it may give the impression that you're angry. Learn to speak distinctly. Careful enunciation is a useful habit to cultivate anyway.

5. You may recall the famous line in a Broadway play "You know I can't hear you when the water's running." Adapt it to include: while the television is on, when the washing machine or the dishwasher is running, or when someone in the same room is carrying on an animated conversation on the telephone. People with hearing loss find it hard to block out sounds while they are straining to hear your words.

6. Don't talk with your back to people with a hearing loss. Even if they can't read your lips accurately when you face them, they will get a better sense of what you're saying.

7. Don't start walking away while you're still talking. Your words will come out as, "I'm going to see if . . ." Frustrating, isn't it?

8. Agree on a signal that you can use in company when your hard-of-hearing spouse is talking too loudly. People with a hearing loss often cannot hear their own voices well enough to judge their own volume level.

9. Don't show annoyance because you must repeat or because the hard-of-hearing person seems to have forgotten something said a few moments ago or even yesterday. He or she probably didn't hear you the first time.

10. Have a heart. Hearing loss is worse for the afflicted person than for anyone else. Consider that you may also have to learn to live with your own hearing loss someday.

Source Unknown

Chapter 8

Spinal Curvature in Osteogenesis Imperfecta

By Heidi C. Glauser
Pittsburgh, Pennsylvania

Scoliosis, or the curvature of the spine, is common in people with OI. According to most of the studies of OI and scoliosis, spinal deformity eventually develops in many people who have mild OI, and in most who have more severe forms.[1] Progressive scoliosis is a potentially severe and disabling problem. In interviewing adults with OI, dialogues typically are centered on back pain due to scoliosis rather than complaints of arm and leg fractures. In addition to back pain, increased disability, and significant deformity, the severest cases of scoliosis could lead to life threatening cardio-pulmonary problems. These complications in turn can add to the immobility of people with OI and accelerate the progression of generalized osteoporosis. Once the spine has developed a significant curvature, it cannot be made entirely straight again. For this reason, it is very important to consult with a surgeon familiar with both scoliosis and OI. Once any degree of curvature occurs, it should be monitored frequently, since it will generally progress.

Spinal Curvature

Spinal curvatures in OI are extremely varied. Sometimes the curve is very slight, and other times it can be extremely pronounced. Single C-shaped curves, bending either left or right are common, as are double or S-shaped curves. Often the spine also twists, or develops outward or inward curvatures.

Curvature of the spine is measured in degrees by using the Cobb method of measurement. First, a series of x-rays are taken by the doctor. Next, two horizontal lines are drawn below the highest vertebra and above the lowest vertebras in the curve.

From these two lines, perpendicular lines are drawn form-ing ninety degree angles which inter-sect with each horizontal line. The resulting new angle or Cobb angle is formed from the intersection of the two perpendicular lines. It is this mea-surement that classi-

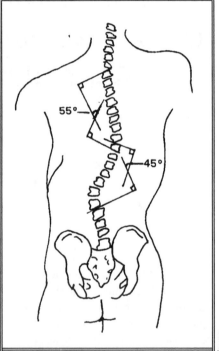

Figure 8-1
Cobb Method of Measuring Spinal Curvature

Artwork by Brian Young

fies the severity of the curve. X-rays from later visits will be compared with the initial X-rays to monitor changes in the curve. (Fig. 8-1)

What Causes Scoliosis in OI?

- **Compression Fractures of the Spine** – Often people with OI experience many compression fractures of the vertebrae. These fractures have been known to occur from any number of activities that jar the spine such as hitting a bump in a wheelchair, falling and landing in a seated position, or driving over a pothole in the road. Sometimes spinal compression fractures are painful, other times they can go unnoticed. Each time one occurs, it may add to the development of scoliosis. It has been reported that these microfractures can also cause damage to the vertebral growth plate.[1]
- **Muscle Strength and Mobility** – Inappropriate wheelchair seating systems can contribute to scoliosis as can prolonged sitting due to lack of ambulation. A discrepancy in the length of the lower extremities or pelvic obliquity can also contribute. Even the slightest imbalance in the vertebrae of the spine can progress quickly to scoliosis. Once the spine does begin to curve, weak muscles in the back are generally not strong enough to pull against the force of the curve, and thus prevent further curvature.

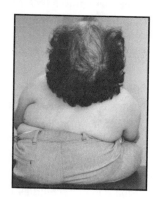

What about Bracing the Back?

In the general population, when scoliosis is detected, the standard treatment to prevent further progression of the curve is to utilize a brace, spinal orthosis, or cast from chin to waist. Unfortunately, this conventional method of preventing further progression of the curvature has not proven to be effective for people with OI. Yong-Hing and MacEwen conducted a survey of seventy-three patients with OI with varying levels of severity. It was determined that the failure rate of treating scoliosis with a Milwaukee type brace was 79 per cent.[3,4] Attempts at bracing people with OI to limit further progression of spinal curvature have been disappointing and usually have had to be abandoned.[5] In some cases, bracing has even been reported to complicate the problem further by causing rib deformities, and by weakening thoracic muscles. Generally the ribs of people with OI are too fragile to transmit corrective forces to the spine. Also, much spinal deformity stems from the vertebrae themselves. It may be reasonable, under carefully controlled circumstances, to consider bracing as an alternative to operative intervention in people with mild forms of OI whose spinal curvatures have not progressed markedly and who have minimal deformity of the wall of the chest.[6] Also, if a limb length discrepancy exists, appropriate orthotics may help to arrest spinal curvature.

Can Electro-Stimulation Help?

Electro-Stimulation, or ESO, is a method of preventing further progression of spinal deformity considered by some. It is rarely recommended for people with OI with severe spinal curvature. Control studies have proven ESO to be an ineffective method of achieving lasting control of spinal curvature.

Spinal Fusion Explained

Spinal fusion is a surgical procedure whereby the vertebrae are fused together. The desired result is a spine where the fused vertebrae behave as a single, solid bone. In recent years, spinal fusion surgery has been performed successfully for many patients with OI. The objective of scoliosis treatment in OI is not so much to correct the curvature but simply to prevent it from getting worse. Although a small degree of correction can be achieved, the primary purpose of spinal fusion is to prevent further deformity, discomfort, and disability. Also, and importantly, fusion of the spine can substantially improve longevity and quality of life.

When to operate?

The monitoring of progressive curvature in people with OI is very important. When to operate should not be determined solely by the age of the patient or by the degree of curvature that exists. Some studies designate 40-50 degrees of spinal curvature as a norm for intervention.

On the other hand, some surgeons, recognizing relentless progression and the eventual difficulties in obtaining correction, may suggest surgical intervention at an earlier stage. In the case of someone with relatively severe OI and progressive curvature, surgical intervention may be recommended when the curve is relatively mild. This approach may prevent the almost certain progression of deformity from developing in the first place, which is preferred over trying to correct the curvature once it has developed. For example, after watching a curve progress from 15 to 30 degrees, a doctor may consider even a 30 degree curve an adequate amount to recommend surgical intervention.[7]

One reason many people consider spinal surgery is because of chronic back pain. Sometimes fusion can reduce or eliminate back pain but it should be noted that in many cases persistent pain continues after the surgery.

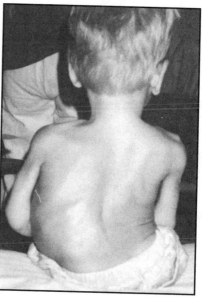

What about Continued Growth and Movement?

It is important to remember that once a portion of the spine is fused, additional height cannot occur in that region of the body. Of course, the legs and the unfused portion of the torso will continue to grow. To some, this consideration alone seems a deterrent when considering spinal fusion for themselves or for their children. But remember, as a severe curve progresses, the growth achieved is rarely upwards, but follows the side-to-side curvature of the spine. Also, for people with OI, once a spine has reached the degree of severity that would warrant a fusion, limited growth can be expected. Actually, after surgery, most people do gain a bit in height. Bending over is slightly restricted following spinal fusion. Although, when a person bends over, most of the movement is at the hip.

How is it done?

There are basically two methods of performing spinal fusion: posteriorly, (through an incision in the back), and both posteriorly and anteriorly, (through the chest and through the back between the lower ribs and hip area). When both anterior and posterior approaches are necessary in order to achieve the most complete stabilization, the curve is first "loosened" by going through the chest to the front of the vertebrae to take out the discs. The discs are important structures in restricting the spinal mobility. The patient is then put in traction, sometimes with a halo around the head. At a second stage surgery, the surgeon goes to the back of the spine and performs the usual spine fusion and instrumentation to hold it.[8] Of course, an anterior/posterior spine fusion involves considerably more risk, and recovery is much more involved. Anterior procedures should not be necessary if spinal deformities are stabilized at an early stage.

Generally, posterior fusion is performed for the majority of people with OI. An incision is made down the length of the spine. Chips of bone, usually obtained from the "bone bank", are sprinkled between the vertebrae of the spine. Then metal instrumentation is used to hold the spine straight while the bone chips fuse with the vertebrae. In some cases, a "glue-like" material called Methylmethacrylate is also used to help secure the instrumentation. There are a number of different instrumentation devices that can be used. The most common types used for people with OI are called the "Harrington Rod", the "Luque" and "Luque-Galveston". The decision of which type of instrumentation is up to the surgeon, and the decision is often made while the patient is on the operating table. The "Harrington Rod" is a straight metal rod with two hooks on each end. After the hooks are attached to the strongest vertebrae at the top and the bottom of the fusion site, the surgeon carefully cranks the mechanism on the rod to achieve maximum straightening. Additional bone chips are placed between the vertebrae and the incision is closed.

In most cases it is recommended that a cast or brace be worn post-operatively to hold the spine in place while the fusion occurs. Sometimes, due to deformities of the chest, a brace or cast cannot be used effectively. If a brace is recommended, a plaster mold can be taken while the patient is still under general anesthesia. From this mold, the brace can be fashioned and made available prior to being discharged from the hospital. The brace can be worn over an undershirt and under a shirt or blouse.

The surgery itself usually takes from three to six hours, depending on the case. After the surgery the waiting begins, with hope that fusion will occur. In a few months, the fusion takes on the consistency of hard chewing gum. After about six to nine months, the fusion should be solid. Although it is rare, occasionally, a spine will not fuse at one, two or three levels. If the surgeon determines that the loss of correction could be affected, sometimes a more local operation is necessary to supplement the larger procedure. After surgery, and the cast or brace is applied, the patient is generally encouraged to sit up and get out of bed within a week or two of surgery.

What Complications Can Occur?

As with any surgery there are risks. This operation has been rated for non-OI populations as follows. On a risk score, where wart removal is a 1 and a heart transplant is 100, it has been calculated that a spine fusion and instrumentation for scoliosis rates 74. Prior to the surgery it is especially important to evaluate pulmonary and respiratory function.[9] Unfortunately, some patients with OI are also very prone to blood loss, so donor blood is required.

The results of spinal fusion in people with OI are satisfactory, although the rate of complications in comparison to the general population, has been fairly high. It is best to consider spinal fusion early because less correction is required and the likelihood of complications is decreased. The most common complication of the surgery is for the hooks of the fixation devise to cause the weak bone to give way and not hold the hooks as it should. Another problem that can develop is that in a

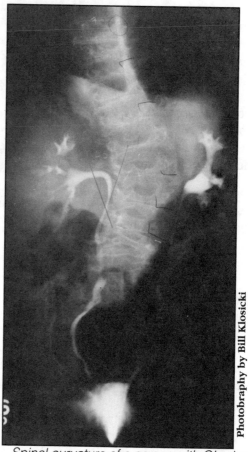

Photobraphy by Bill Klosicki

Spinal curvature of a person with OI prior to spinal fusion surgery.

local area, full fusion does not occur, but, instead, a fibrous band simply connects two bony areas resulting in an incomplete fusion, and possibly the need for an additional surgery.

The possible risks of spinal surgery include paralysis, infection, cardiac arrest, pneumonia, stress ulcers, kidney shutdown, blood transfusion reactions, hepatitis, and so forth. All of these risks are small, but nevertheless do exist.

What about Pain and Recovery?

Some people with OI have reported spinal fusion surgery as being less painful than rodding surgeries for arms or legs. The incision is generally quite large, and should be monitored for infection and proper healing. It is usually necessary for the person to lay flat in bed for ten to fourteen days. In the hospital most patients request Patient Controlled Anesthesia, or PCAs, to control post-surgery pain.

After surgery, the patient is required to wear a brace or cast for nine months to a year. A brace naturally is preferable to the person with OI, and is recommended with strict instructions for its removal. The "clam shell" type brace with Velcro side closures is most convenient.

Photobraphy by Bill Klosicki

View of post-surgery spinal fusion. The Cotrel-Dubousset Instrumentation rod shown stabilizes the curvature and prevents further progression of the scoliosis.

It should be noted that stabilization of a spinal curve cannot be expected to improve or hinder a person's ability to walk.

Daily Living Following Spinal Fusion Surgery

Initially, the person, when turned, must be "log rolled." This means that the entire body must roll as a unit. The brace helps in this.

Sponge baths are recommended for about one month. At that point, if possible, the person can then take the brace off for bathing, assuring that he or she not sit, or bear weight on the spine without the brace. If possible the person must be lifted flat into and out of the bathtub. Another alternative is to wear the brace into the bathtub. In this case, outer clothing is removed, but the brace and undershirt remain on. After the bath, and while laying flat, the person removes the brace and wet undershirt, dries the brace with a towel, and replaces the wet undershirt with a dry one.

Recreational pursuits, including swimming, are to be encouraged provided the person is extremely cautious in avoiding falls, jarring, or accidents during the period of recovery.

School-aged children who undergo spinal fusion surgery sometimes establish temporary home tutoring during their recovery period. At the point when sitting can be resumed, the child can then return to school, monitoring closely the amount of time in any given position for discomfort, fatigue, or muscle spasms.

Summary

Scoliosis is a very common and troubling complication of osteogenesis imperfecta. It is extremely important that people with OI receive regular orthopaedic monitoring of any progression of spinal curvature. In most cases early surgical intervention is recommended. Stabilization and the prevention of further curvature is the goal of spinal fusion surgery, not correction of an existing curve. Spinal fusion surgery for people with OI is generally successful.

Endnotes

1. Hanscom, D., Winter, R., Lutter, L., Lonstein, J., Bloom, B., Bradford, D., ""Osteogenesis Imperfecta", The Journal of Bone and Joint Surgery, Vol. 74-A, No. 4, 598-615 (Apr. 1992) 612.
2. Norimatsu, H., Tadashi, M., Takahashi, H., The Development of Spinal Deformities in Osteogenesis Imperfecta, Clinical Orthopedics, 162: 20-25. 1982, 23.
3. Ibid., 23.
4. Benson, D., Donaldson, D., and Millar, E., The Spine in Osteogenesis Imperfecta., Clinical Orthopedics, 60-A: 925-929, Oct. 1978.

5. **Yong-Hing, K., MacEwen, G. D.**, *Scoliosis associated with osteogenesis imperfecta: Results of treatment, Journal of Bone and Joint Surgery, 64B:36, 1982.*.

6. **Cristofaro, R., Hoek, K., Bonnett, C., Brown, J.**, *Operative Treatment of Spine Deformity in Osteogenesis Imperfecta, Clinical Orthopedics, 139: 40-48. 1979, 47.*

7. **Hanscom**, *et al., 613.*

8. *Oppenheim, W.L., UCLA Medical Center, (personal communication, March 11, 1994)*

9. **Bleck, E., Rinsky, L., Gamble, J.**, *The Scoliosis Program, Children's Hospital at Stanford, pamphlet, 4.*

10. **Ibid.**, *5.*

Chapter 9

Pain Control Alternatives for People with OI

by **Lawrence C. Vogel, M.D.**
Director of Pediatrics
Shriners Hospitals for Crippled Children, Chicago Unit

"Pain is soul destroying. No patient should have to endure intense pain unnecessarily. The quality of mercy is essential to the practice of medicine; here, of all places, it should not be strained." Marcia Angell, M.D. (N. Engl J Med; 306:98-99).

Pain is a very unpleasant experience which deserves aggressive management in a timely and safe manner. Too often, physicians and nurses are reluctant to adequately treat pain because of fear of complications, such as drowsiness or respiratory depression or unfounded concerns of addiction. People may also be hesitant to request adequate pain relief because of similar concerns, fear of discomfort of intramuscular injections (shots), and being labeled as a bad patient and a wimp ("no pain, no gain").

Relieving pain should be a top priority for health care workers, people with OI, and their families. Pain management should be a comprehensive program which includes a combination of medicines and non-pharmacological measures, such as visualization and relaxation techniques. It should involve continuing input from an interdisciplinary team which may include pediatricians, internists, orthopedic surgeons, anesthesiologists, psychiatrists, psychologists, nurses, physical, occupational, or recreation therapists, child life specialists, and pharmacists. People with OI and their families must be integral members of the interdisciplinary team. A pain management program should be initiated prior to painful events, if possible, and must include continued monitoring of effectiveness and safety, and appropriate adjustments.

What is Pain?

The International Association for the Study of Pain defines pain as "an unpleasant sensory and emotional experience associated with actual or potential tissue damage, or described in terms of such damage." Qualitative and quantitative aspects of pain vary greatly between different individuals and also for the same person depending upon dynamic physical and psychological factors. As an example, the intensity and duration of pain associated with stubbing your toe can vary greatly depending upon whether you've just won the state lottery or just written out a check to the IRS.

Pain originates when nerve endings, such as those found in skin or bone, are irritated by stimuli such as a fractured bone. The impulse travels through the nerve, up the spinal cord and finally to the brain. Our brains process these signals based upon past experiences with pain, our emotional and psychological state, and thought assessment. The end result is our perception of pain which includes intensity, duration, and the quality or characteristics of pain, such as dull, sharp, cramping, or radiating. If pain is not adequately treated or the originating painful stimulus is not removed, the transmission of pain impulses to our brain occurs more readily. This phenomenon explains why it is easier to prevent pain than to chase it. For example, after orthopedic surgery on a leg, it takes less medicine and is more effective to prevent the associated pain of initially bearing weight by administering medication prior to therapy than to try to chase worsening pain with medication after physical therapy is initiated.

Pain is not a disease in itself. Pain is a symptom, a warning that something is wrong. When we experience pain, we try to identify and relieve or remove the cause if possible. A person may take medication and seek medical attention to resolve the underlying causes and receive further symptomatic treatment of the pain.

People manifest pain in a number of ways, both verbally and non-verbally. They may cry, yell out in pain, or inform the nurse or physician that something hurts and and requires pain medication. Nonverbal responses to pain include elevated heart rate and blood pressure and immobilization of an injured part in order to avoid pain on motion. The responses to pain may not always be beneficial. One example of this is the difficulty of taking a deep breath after a spine fusion because of pain experienced. This avoidance of pain may result in collapse of portions of the lung or pneumonia.

Pain Assessment

There are a number of methods available to quantify the amount of pain that you are experiencing. These pain intensity scales rate pain from no pain to the worst possible pain and use numbers, words, or pictures to depict the degree of pain. These pain scales are very useful in establishing, monitoring, and modifying pain management programs and are most commonly used in the post-operative period.

In addition, a person with OI should let the doctor, nurse, or other health care workers know the severity of the pain and his or her response to current pain treatment. A self-report about the severity of the pain is the single most important information available to the doctor or nurse in management of the pain. In addition, a person's past experiences with pain and its treatment are very important in planning a successful pain management program.

Advantages of Effective Pain Management

It has been clearly demonstrated that people who receive adequate pain management postoperatively experience fewer complications, have decreased hospital stays, and reduced hospital costs. Adequate pain control allows for decreased immobilization, improved postoperative activities, and increased participation in physical and occupational therapy. This decreases the incidence of blood clots. It also improves deep breathing exercises and the ability to cough, and this reduces pulmonary complications, such as pneumonia and the collapse of portions of the lung.

Equally as important, effective pain management results in

increased satisfaction and less anxiety the next time you are exposed to painful situations. Lastly, as health care professionals, we find great satisfaction in participating in one of our most noble and time-honored activities of relieving pain and suffering.

Non-pharmacological Symptomatic Care

Non-pharmacological symptomatic measures are particularly ideal because they are not costly, are easily learned, have few side effects, can usually be self-administered at home or in a health care setting, are well accepted, and are usually beneficial. Individuals with OI and their families quickly learn that immobilization or splinting of a fractured extremity significantly relieves pain. Ice and elevation decrease swelling and subsequent discomfort during the first few days after an injury or surgery. Massage and heat may also be beneficial, especially when muscle tightness or spasms are present. TENS or Transcutaneous Electrical Nerve Stimulation may also be beneficial in alleviating pain.

Behavioral and cognitive maneuvers such as relaxation, distraction, imagery, and hypnosis are very useful components of pain management. Music assisted relaxation has been proven to be beneficial. Relaxation can also be affected by a jaw relaxation technique or slow rhythmic breathing. Distraction can be accomplished by watching TV, reading a book, talking on the telephone, or playing an age-appropriate game. Imagery or visualization can simply consist of picturing a warm and sunny beach. More complex imagery, hypnosis, and biofeedback require greater professional involvement. Regardless of age, when we are hurting we want familiar people and things near us. This may include our favorite "blankie," toy, or loved one's hand holding ours.

A pain management center may be helpful for people with OI who suffer from chronic pain. There, specialists can provide education and instruction for various techniques including massage therapy, relaxation, visualization, hydrotherapy. Many of these techniques are not "scientifically proven" treatments and no definitive claims can be made about their effectiveness. Many people report substantial beneficial results from these practices, however, and many have merit if used as an adjunct to and not a substitute for a sound medically directed program.

Pain can also be more readily controlled if we are well informed about surgical procedures, the expected sequence of events and associated pain, and the plan to alleviate pain and anxiety. Children undergoing surgeries or painful procedures similarly must be well informed in a developmentally appropriate manner.

Medications

Medications are the mainstay of management of pain. To be most effective in alleviating pain, medications should be administered before pain appears and certainly before it worsens. Pain medications should be administered prior to painful procedures or before the performance of an activity that may be painful, such as deep breathing exercises after a spine fusion. As stated earlier, it is best to prevent pain rather than chase it. Pain is best prevented or treated by providing pain medication on a continuous or around the clock basis rather than as needed. Pain medications should be administered in an acceptable manner that is less uncomfortable than the pain itself. Ideally, they should be administered orally, intravenously, or under the tongue. Medications taken orally are generally the least expensive and most convenient alternative. Intramuscular injections are painful and should be a last resort.

Mild to moderate pain can usually be managed with non-steroidal

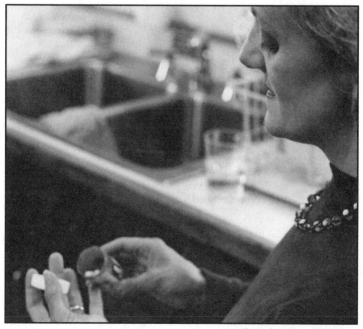

Photo by Laura Vinchesi

anti-inflammatory drugs (NSAIDs). These include medications such as aspirin, ibuprofen, (Motrin, Advil, Nuprin), choline magnesium trisalicylate, (Trilisate), and naproxen, (Naprosyn, Anaprox). The NSAIDs are given orally and may be given as needed for mild pain or around the clock for moderate pain. The main side effects of NSAIDs are gastric irritation which ranges from an upset stomach to a bleeding ulcer, and interference with coagulation, resulting in a tendency to bleed or bruise. Gastric side effects can be minimized by administering NSAIDs with a meal. NSAIDs affect coagulation by interfering with a clotting factor of the blood. This is seen most commonly with aspirin but can be seen with most other NSAIDs. Because there is some evidence that people with OI have a coagulation disorder related to platelet dysfunction, we do not recommend use of NSAIDs preoperatively. In addition, there is concern that NSAIDs may interfere with bone formation, so we generally avoid this class of drugs in people who have healing bones subsequent to surgery or a fracture.

Ketorolac is a new NSAID which can be administered intramuscularly and may be as effective as narcotics. Although only approved for intramuscular or oral use, it is frequently used intravenously. However, Ketorolac would have limited use in individuals with OI because of the potential interference with bone healing.

Acetaminophen, (Tylenol), is similar to NSAID in its analgesic and ability to help reduce fever, but it does not have anti-inflammatory activity. It is readily available, relatively free of side effects and can be administered orally or as a rectal suppository.

For moderate to severe pain, narcotics are usually needed. Morphine is the standard to which other narcotics (opioids) are compared. Narcotics vary in their potency and the route by which they may be administered. Side effects are similar for all of the narcotics and range from constipation, urinary retention, nausea and vomiting, to drowsiness and respiratory depression.

A persisting and unfounded fear about narcotics is its addicting potential when used for the management of acute pain. Addiction is extremely unlikely to develop after a person with no prior drug abuse history use opioids for acute pain. When narcotics are used for more than several weeks for persistent pain, a person may require larger doses to attain the same degree of pain relief. This represents tolerance and not addiction. All narcotics should be administered under close supervision of a qualified professional.

For severe pain and in the immediate postoperative period,

narcotics are usually administered intravenously. Using "patient controlled analgesia" (PCA), a patient seven years or older can self-administer a narcotic such as morphine intravenously. The patient controls the PCA with a button which, when pressed, delivers a preset amount of morphine. The frequency for which the intermittent doses can be administered and the maximum amount of narcotic administered within a four hour period are also preset. For optimal effectiveness, the person needs to be educated in the appropriate use of PCA. This includes pushing the button when pain begins or is expected to occur. In order to provide a constant background of analgesia and supplement PCA, a low dose of a narcotic can be infused continuously. This is called "PCA plus" and helps to avoid a person from waking up in severe pain because they were sleeping and unable to press their PCA button. Continuous intravenous administration of narcotics may be useful in children who are developmentally too young for PCA or for anyone not capable of utilizing PCA.

When people are able to take medications orally, there are a variety of narcotics, alone or in combination with acetaminophen, that are effective in moderate to moderately severe pain. Codeine, which is usually combined with acetaminophen, (Tylenol with codeine), is frequently used and is very effective. Hydrocodone with acetaminophen (Vicodin) is another commonly used combination and may provide relief for more severe pain compared to acetaminophen with codeine. Other narcotics that can be given orally include morphine, methadone, oxycodone with acetaminophen (Percocet), hydromophone (Dilaudid), levorphanol (Levo-Dromoran), and propoxyphene with acetaminophen, (Darvocet-N). The use of fetanyl lollipops may be useful as a preoperative medication for young children.

Frequently, when people are in pain, they are also experiencing some degree of anxiety which usually increases the impact of the pain. When anxiety is a major contributor of the discomfort that a person in pain is experiencing, medications that reduce anxiety, such as anxiolytics, may be beneficial. Midazolam (Versed) or diazepam (Valium) are two of the most commonly used anxiolytics. In addition, Valium has the added advantage of being a muscle relaxant which is beneficial to many people with OI after orthopedic surgery. The major problem with the use of anxiolytics is respiratory depression that is particularly common when anxiolytics are administered concurrently with narcotics.

The use of different medications, different routes of administration, as well as non-pharmacological measures can result in a cooperative response in which the end result is better than that expected from merely adding together the effects of each individual modality. An example would be the postoperative administration of around the clock oral or rectal acetaminophen, morphine administered via PCA along with continuous infusion, (PCA plus), and relaxation exercises and imagery. This program could be further augmented with epidurally administered local anesthetics in order to decrease the amount of morphine administered intravenously.

Conscious Sedation

When a person is undergoing painful therapeutic or diagnostic procedures, the use of medications to prevent or reduce pain, discomfort or anxiety may be indicated. This type of intervention is called conscious sedation because you remain easily arousable, responsive to verbal stimuli, and maintain your protective airway reflexes. A combination of a narcotic and an anxiolytic, (Fentanyl and Versed administered IV), may be used for a painful procedure; whereas, chloral hydrate given orally, a sedative, may be the most appropriate medication for a non-painful radiological procedure such as a MRI (magnetic resonance imaging). The main problem with conscious sedation is the potential for the person to inadvertently progress to deep sedation with loss of protective airway reflexes and the need for ventilatory support. Whenever a patient is provided with conscious sedation, he must be monitored very closely by a qualified health care worker for whom this is their sole responsibility.

Conclusion

Pain is no longer an acceptable alternative for any individual with OI. There are a multitude of measures available that can alleviate pain in a relatively safe manner and result in better outcomes. It is a joint effort for the person, the family, and health care providers to assure that pain is minimized. Open communication among all involved parties is paramount for success in these endeavors.

For those interested in further information about pain management, the U.S. Department of Health and Human Services has published an excellent monograph entitled: Clinical Practice Guidelines. Acute Pain Management: Operative or Medical Procedures and Trauma (1992). They have also published a brochure entitled "Pain Control After Surgery: A Patient's Guide." For copies call 1-800-358-9295.

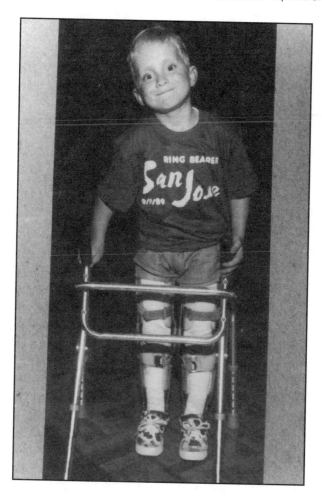

Chapter 10

Making Educated Surgical Decisions about Rodding

By Edward A. Millar, MD and Peter Smith, MD
Shrine Hospital, Chicago Unit, Chicago, Illinois

The goal of the orthopedic surgeon is to maximize function and to minimize deformity for people with OI. Since OI is a variable disorder, there is not one particular solution to the problems encountered by all people with OI. Doctors should avoid trying to treat OI as though using a cookbook. They should keep in mind the individuality of the patient and the uniqueness of each case. Not everyone with a fracture needs to be in a cast for six weeks, and by the same token, not everyone with OI needs intramedullary rods.

The Purpose of Rodding

The purpose of rodding surgery is to achieve a functional goal – such as to stand and transfer , or to improve ambulating ability, or decrease fracture numbers in a limb which has had

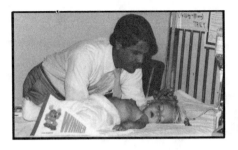

numerous re-fractures. When fractures do occur, the rod keeps the bone fragments in position and generally hastens the healing process. Rodding may also allow the person to be more active after a fracture, and to avoid prolonged periods of casting and inactivity. This, in turn, can help break cycles of inactivity leading to fractures.

Ambulation probably should not be the principle goal of surgery because ability to walk, in large part, is determined by many factors including the severity of the OI, the potential for sufficient muscle development, the size of the bone, the frequency and severity of fractures, and the severity of deformities.

Considerations

Intramedullary rodding is usually indicated when either severe deformities exist or repeated fractures occur. The thigh bone, or femur, and lower leg bone, or tibia, most commonly require rodding. On occasions, rods may be used in the upper arm bone, or humerus, and less frequently in the bones of the forearms.

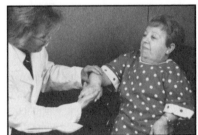

Obviously, whenever the idea of surgery is entertained, there are risks and benefits to be considered. The benefits of successful rodding are:

- Prevention of fractures
- Straightening the deformities in the long bones
- Increasing the feasibility of weight-bearing and bracing
- Improving function and perhaps mobility

When to perform rodding surgery

While the rodding procedure has been performed on children as young as 3 months, the timing of the surgery is usually based on when the child has reached functional gross development, such as pulling to stand or beginning to walk. The age can vary in the child's development. Occasionally the surgeon will elect to operate on two bones at one sitting, but if the surgery is extensive, it is usually best to operate on a single bone.

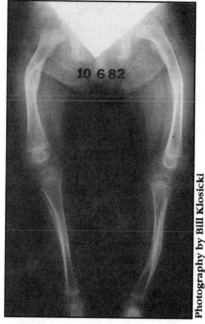

Methods

A procedure such as rodding is made possible by the nature of the long bones. Simply put, the bone is made up of a hollow tube, the ends of which are closed off by solid blocks of bone near the joints which contain the growth plates. In OI, it is this slender, hollow tube portion of the bone which often bows and breaks. The rodding operation consists of cutting through the muscle and other soft tissues to expose the long bone shaft. At areas where there has been a fracture or the bone is bent, the bone is cut and

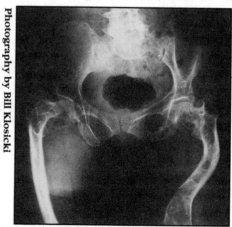

X-ray views of bowed femurs (thigh bones) of two children with OI showing excessive, but not uncommon deformities that frequently suggest the need for rodding.

realigned. Rarely is the long shaft of bone totally removed from the leg.
A steel rod of proper length is then threaded through the bone segments

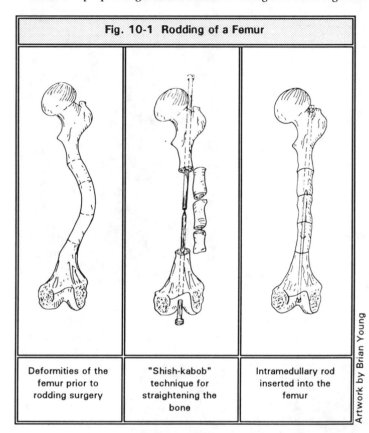

Fig. 10-1 Rodding of a Femur

| Deformities of the femur prior to rodding surgery | "Shish-kabob" technique for straightening the bone | Intramedullary rod inserted into the femur |

Artwork by Brian Young

to make a straight bone. The long shaft of bone is broken up into short
segments and strung onto the rod like elongated beads, much like a
shish-kabob. The number of segments into which the bone must be cut
depends on the degree of curvature in the bone prior to surgery. (Fig.
10-1)

Another dimension that must be considered is that the bones of
the person with OI, although they may appear round on the X-ray and
able to accept a rod, are sometimes flat and thin when seen in another
dimension.

After the bone segments are threaded onto the rod, the free end
of the rod is anchored into the opposite joint and the limb is then
supported in a cast or splint until these segments of bone grow together
in about four to eight weeks.

It is sometimes possible to thread a rod through the bone without making an extensive incision. With the aid of a portable X-ray machine, we can sometimes rod a femur fracture by passing the rod through the skin in the hip area, or a tibia fracture by passing the rod through the heel. If this is possible, it is preferable because it takes a shorter time to heal and is less traumatic to the soft tissues.

Many people ask how the body tolerates rodding surgery when the marrow of the bone is violated. Rest assured that the bone contains sufficient marrow to allow a rod to pass through without compromising its integrity.

Plates and Screws

Plates and screws are popularly used in adult orthopedics. These stabilize the fracture and keep the bone in alignment so that adequate healing can take place. Plates and screws are most often used to aid in the healing of hip fractures in adults who have fairly good bone. They can work initially in people with OI, but tend not to work very well in the long run. The problem is that fractures tend to occur at the top and bottom of the plate and also the plate tends to move around. In addition, in OI bone the screws eventually loosen and come out. Generally, plates and screws are not recommended for a child, but there may be isolated circumstances where this is the best treatment method.

Types of rods

Rods are made in various lengths and thicknesses, and can be ordered according to the estimated size of the bone. The length and diameter depend on the size of the bone to be rodded. Generally, these rods should be thinner in diameter than the thick heavy rods commonly used by orthopedists in adult trauma cases.

There are basically two types of rods used in people with OI.

- **Non-extensible Rods** – The non-extensible rods looks very much like a large straight pin. It is very versatile, easy to fashion to the individual, and it's relatively easy to insert. You can often insert it percutaneously, or through the skin without a large incision. One complication of the non-extensible rod is that sometimes the bones grow beyond the length of the rod. Parts of bone then become unsupported, the rod can begin to migrate, and the bone sometimes bows away from the rod. If this occurs, the rod can begin to protrude from the skin, and the likelihood of fractures will increase. It is common for non-extensible rods to require replacement in children who are growing fairly rapidly. The average time a non-extensible rod functions is two years.

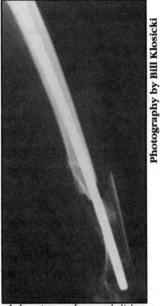

A fracture of an adult lower leg (tibia) is stabilized by an intramedullary rod.

Photography by Bill Klosicki

- **Telescoping Intramedullary Rods** – An alternative rod, used frequently in people with OI, is the telescoping or elongating rod. It is a two-piece rod, fashioned basically as a rod within a rod. It can be roughly described as a straight pin inside a straw. It has a button at either end and it expands like a trombone as the bone grows. One advantage to the telescoping rod is that due to its ability to grow with the child, it needs to be replaced less frequently. A disadvantage is that the extensible rods may fail to extend, or the button can come off, or they may bend because they're more malleable.

Telescoping rods are used most often on the thigh bone (femur) and extend across the growth plate at the knee. They work especially well in the larger child. A smaller child may get irritated where the end of the rod projects into the knee joint. However, this irritation usually subsides with growth. Such a rod is difficult to use in the tibia, or lower leg bone, since there is little room for the end of the rod in the ankle joint

The type of rod used in an individual case depends on several factors. Much of the decision actually depends on the surgeon's comfort and familiarity with a particular rod. Studies have shown that complications resulting from the use of the non-extensible rod and the extensible rod are equal and the rate of re-operation required for both rods is similar.

• **Other Rods** – New rods are being developed constantly. Other rods that are now being used are the thinner and more flexible Rush and Enders rods.

Arms

Because the upper extremities do not bear as much weight and have less tendency to fracture, they generally require less surgical intervention. Also, any bowing that may occur in the arm is less likely to interfere with the function of the limb. Surgery to solely improve cosmetic appearance is not advisable.

Surgery on upper extremities is useful in situations where there are repetitive fractures of the arms. If the bone repeatedly breaks after a cast is removed, sometimes the cycle can be broken by placing a rod in one of the arm bones.

Legs

Intramedullary rodding surgery is most useful in the lower extremities. As children begin to pull themselves up and bear weight on the legs, rodding surgery can help to prevent progressive bowing deformities and recurrent fractures. If significant deformities already exist when the child begins to stand, there is a potential for fractures to occur. The bowing deformity which predisposes to fracture is frequently difficult to correct with casting alone.

In the tibia, or shin bone, there's a characteristic bowing in many children with OI. Sometimes this can be accommodated with a brace and sometimes it cannot. Other times the bowed area becomes progressively more painful and X-rays reveal an area where fractures are occurring repeatedly. In this circumstance it's useful to do rodding as well.

Anesthesia

Many persons with OI react badly to certain types of anesthesia. Certain medications, such as atropine, need to be avoided. Usually the problems that occur, such as nausea, elevated temperature, and excessive bleeding, can be controlled by the anesthesiologist. Complications from anesthesia must be carefully monitored and alternative medication considered.

Complications

With any type of surgery there can be complications. Excessive bleeding and infections have occurred, although they are actually very rare in OI. Infections and failure of the bone to become solid are very rare.

Other complications with the rods include technical difficulties placing the rod, and occasionally the malfunction of a rod, such as the button end of the rods breaking off. Another complication is the tendency for the rods to migrate, and back out of the bone.

Remember that bone is living tissue which is constantly remolding. With growth, the long portion of the bone may again gradually bow until the end of the rod begins to protrude through the skin, requiring a change of the rod. Usually the second operation does not require as much surgery as the first one.

Bones can refracture as they outgrow the rods. Where repeated operations are required, the bone may become quite thin, requiring a delay in additional surgery in anticipation of the bone to grow sufficiently to accommodate the proper size rod. On the other hand, very large rods may shield the bone from stress and cause it to waste away. This situation can generally be prevented by using thinner, more flexible rods.

The one question quite naturally asked often, is, "How safe an operation is intramedullary rodding?" The operation is one of major proportions, yet people with OI tolerate it very well.

Summary

Our knowledge about successful orthopaedic treatment of people with OI improves every year. We feel assured that methods in orthopaedic surgery are continually improving as we strive to make life better for people with OI.

Chapter 11

Further Complications of OI

by Heidi C. Glauser
Pittsburgh, Pennsylvania

Growth Deficiency

Growth deficiency is the most prevalent secondary feature of OI. All individuals with type III OI have severe growth deficiency; most individuals with moderate OI will be shorter than standard growth curves and even those with type I OI may be shorter than unaffected family members. Although fractures may be associated with disproportionate growth, there is no clear relationship between fracture number and growth deficiency. Fractures involving the growth plate are relatively uncommon.

At the National Institutes of Health, Dr. Joan Marini and colleagues are examining the status of hormones related to growth in OI children. Findings suggest subtle abnormalities of the growth hormone-somatomedin axis in some children, with resistance to growth hormone action. A treatment trial of growth hormone for types I, IV and III OI is being conducted. Both changes in growth rate and effect on bone quality are being investigated. Administration of growth hormone appears to increase growth rates in some children during short term administration. However, the effect on final stature is unknown.

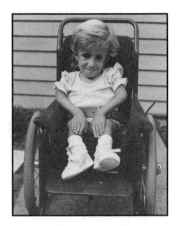

Basilar Impression

Basilar impression, or BI, is compression of the base of the skull and aportion of the brain or spinal cord with resultant neurological complications. The frequency of BI is unknown but appears to affect people with OI type III or OI type IV. Initial symptoms can include:

- Dizziness
- Neck extension causing giddiness
- Exaggeration of the reflexes
- Increased resistance of muscles to passive stretching
- A flickering of the eyes when looking down[2]

Complications resulting from basilar impression can be extremely debilitating, and at the first appearance of symptoms, people with OI should seek medical care.[3]

Hydrocephalus

Sometimes children with OI may be thought to have a larger head size than expected and the question of hydrocephalus may be raised. Hydrocephalus is characterized by an abnormal increase of pressure in the fluid in the central portion of the brain causing enlargement of the head. A recent study by Tsipouras,et al. found that these children did not have hydrocephalus. Some children with OI have large heads and ventricular dilatation but the pressure is not increased. The expansion probably occurs because the bone is soft.[6]

Hyperplastic Callus Formation

Hyperplastic callus formation, or an overgrowth of repair tissue around fractures occurs in a very small number of people with OI. This phenomenon may suggest to the examining physician a malignant cancer of the bone. In a study by Keessen and collegues, two teenagers with OI developed hyperplastic callus on the upper margin of the hip bone. The symptoms included: severe swelling and pain in the upper leg and buttock region. They were both treated with indomethacin, a non-steroidal drug which reduces swelling and eases pain.[4]

Anesthetic Considerations

People with OI are at a greater risk than the general population for a number of complications during anesthesia. Sometimes the mobility of the neck and jaw in a person with OI is restricted by deformity. Also chest and rib deformities may restrict the ability to breathe. Other associated complications such as problems with the teeth, cleft palate, joint stiffness, and heart valve disease may increase the hazards of anesthesia. Of course, anesthesiologists must take into account the susceptibility of people with OI to fracture when moving or rolling the patient with OI.

Another complication reported to be a relatively common anesthetic consideration for OI is hyperthermia, or an increase in body temperature. It has been stated that the hyperthermia during and after anesthesia in patients with OI does not progress to malignant hyperthermia, a particularly severe form of the condition. People with OI and parents of children with OI could suggest the following article as

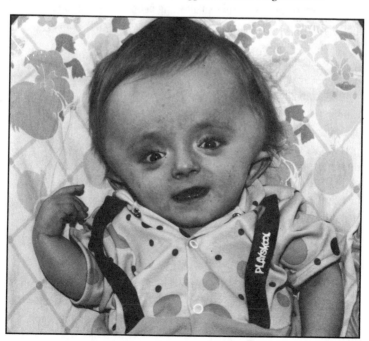

recommended reading for their anesthesiologist prior to surgery.[5]

C. Anthony Ryan, Abdullah S. Al-Ghamdi, Michael Gayle, and Neil N. Finer, Osteogenesis Imperfecta and Hyperthermia, *Anesthesia and Analgesia*, 68:(6):881-4, 1989 Jun.

Non-union of Fractures

After a fracture occurs, the bone normally begins the healing process right away. Usually, the bone will knit itself back together, and the fracture becomes healed. Sometimes in people with OI, especially when there is a pattern of repeated fractures and deformity at one site, the healing process stops before bony continuity is restored.[7] Although non-unions are generally painless, they can lead to a marked decrease in functional ability and sometimes a discrepancy in limb length. The customary treatment for non-union is to operate on the site that will not heal. Generally the disjoined portion of the bone is removed, a intramedullary rod is inserted, and bone-grafting is performed.[8]

Respiratory Complications of OI

Serious respiratory complications are likely to affect individuals with severe forms of OI. Additionally, individuals with less severe forms of OI may have respiratory complications due to progressive scoliosis. The primary respiratory problem affecting people with OI is a loss of lung capacity. To a variable extent, the lungs are trapped in an abnormal chest wall due to distorted ribs or spinal curvature. This abnormality can limit the amount of air a person can inhale during a forceful effort. For normal activities, and particularly when well, this loss of lung capacity does not cause discomfort in

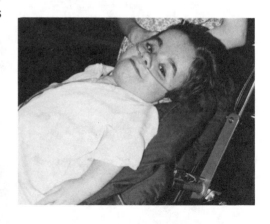

daily living. Strenuous activity and respiratory infection, however, can magnify a reduced lung capacity in the form of shortness of breath. The limited amount of respiratory reserve make additional lung function difficult.

Normally, a modest reduction in respiratory capacity does not affect the lung's ability to perform its primary task; extracting oxygen from air and releasing carbon dioxide on exhalation. When a marked reduction in lung capacity occurs, however, normal oxygenation may not be possible and supplementation of oxygen by a nasal catheter or mask may be necessary to perform daily activities comfortably. Should the reduction in lung capacity become severe, assisted breathing, particularly during sleep, can be enormously successful in improving respiratory performance during daytime activities.

If the limited lung capacity common in advanced scoliosis, or the severe forms of OI, is coupled with additional respiratory disease, respiratory function may become severely, albeit temporarily, impaired. Pneumonia, bronchitis, and asthma are common problems that may be particularly troublesome, but are nonetheless manageable. Finally, respiratory function can be easily defined by a few simple tests. These tests can be helpful and should be considered by some people with OI to reveal changes in lung capacity over time, define the risks of major surgery, and/or demonstrate recovery during acute illness.[9]

Endnotes

1. **Marini, J.C., Bordenick, S., Heavner, G., Rose, S. Hintz, R., Rosenfeld, R. Chrousos, G.**, *The Growth Hormone and Somatomedin Axis in Short Children with Osteogenesis Imperfecta, Journal of Clinical Endrocrinology and Metabolism., 76:1, 1993.*

2. **Turner, A.M., Sillence, D.O.**, *Craniocervical Complications of Osteogenesis Imperfecta. IV International Conference on Osteogenesis Imperfecta - Abstracts. Pavia, Italy, 1990.*

3. **Harkey, H.L., Crockard, H.A., Stevens, J.M., Smith, R., Ransford, A.O.**, *The Operative Management of Basilar Impression in Osteogenesis Imperfecta. Neurosurgery. 27:5, 782-785, 1990.*

4. **Keessen, W., Vanpaemel, L., Breslau-Siderius, R., Engelbert, S., Geelen, P., Kramer,** *Department of Orthopaedics, Physical Therapy, Pediatrics, Radiology, Wilhemina Children's Hospital and Clinical Genetics Center, Utrecht State University, Fourth International Conference on OI - Abstracts, 1993.*

5. **Ryan, C.A., Al-Ghamdi, A.S., Gayle, M., Finer, N.N.**, *Osteogenesis Imperfecta and Hyperthermia, Anesthesia and Analgesia, 68(6):881-4, 1989 Jun.*

6. **Tsipouras, P., M.D., Barabas, G., M.D., Matthews, W.S., Ph.D.**, *Neurologic Correlates of Osteogenesis Imperfecta, Archive of Neurology, 43:150-152, 1986.*

7. **Brighton, C.T.**, *The Semi-Invasive Method of Treating Nonunion with Direct Current, Clinical Orthopaedics Clinics, North America, 15:33-45, 1984.*

8. **Gamble, J.G., Rinsky, M.D., Studwick J., Bleck, E.E.**, *Non-union of Fractures in Children Who Have Osteogenesis Imperfecta, Journal of Bone and Joint Surgery, 70-A, No. 3, March 1988.*

9. **Kuracheck, Steve M.D.** *Personal communication, May 1994.*

Chapter 12

Thoughts about Research and the Medical Management of OI Through the Years

by Heidi C. Glauser
Pittsburgh, Pennsylvania

Over the years, practitioners, investigators, and people with OI have tried many different methods to treat, eliminate, or improve the symptoms of the disabling condition called osteogenesis imperfecta. A brief scan of medical reports about treatments for OI would reveal a myriad of modalities that have been tried, and have actually been "proven successful." Publications contain over 55 articles about mineral and mineral compound treatments, over 21 reports of vitamin treatments, over nine reports of diets that have been tried, and multitudes of other concoctions including bone marrow, adrenaline, and radiation. Within all this literature about possible methods of treatment for OI, the majority of the reports, (70%), state that the treatment under study is beneficial for people with OI. Only 19% state that no improvement was observed, and 10% are inconclusive.[1] (Figure 12-1) So then, why are all these beneficial treatments not being utilized? This chapter will briefly discuss a few of the treatments of OI that have been studied, and the difficulties encountered in the study of OI.

The first recorded report of improvement in a patient with OI was reported in the American Journal of Medical Science in 1897 by J.P. Griffith. He stated that a person with OI had improved health following treatment with phosphorus, cod liver oil, fresh air and exercise.[2] Since then there have been increasing numbers of articles.

It is important to distinguish the different types of studies that are conducted in order to obtain an objective outlook on the OI research that has been reported. The following three hypothetical cases will clarify part of the reason why the findings of so many of the OI studies are erroneous or inconclusive.

Case 1:

Josh, a child with severe OI, has a pediatrician, who is convinced that a certain medication would curb the fracture rate of his patient. Josh undergoes the prescribed treatment, and, his fracture rate drops by 50%. The doctor writes up his findings, and reports that this medication proved to be helpful to Josh.

Case 2:

An investigator recruits eight people with OI to participate in a study he is conducting. He records their bone density at the onset, and then administers high doses of a certain vitamin. After a two year period, he notes a slight increase in the bone density of his patients. His concluding report is positive.

Case 3:

Dr. Smart, is affiliated with a team of experienced investigators. He contacts a group of 25 people with OI to participate in his study. He also secures the services of an adequate control group, (more people with OI), making it possible to differentiate any possible effect due to the treatment, from the expected decrease in fractures rate with age. He follows the progress of all these people for four years. His findings, at the conclusion of the study, are considered valid.

After reviewing the above three hypothetical cases, a problem should be evident. Although OI has been studied quite extensively through the years, the results reported, are often inaccurate or inconclusive due to a number of factors. First, how and where can an investigator find a large number of people with OI to participate in a study? Since there are relatively few people with OI in any one geographical area, the difficulty and expense incurred in recruiting and accessing standardized information from them must be considered. It is also important to recognize that many of the positive results of these studies are based upon the clinical changes that occur in people with OI. In other words, if the fracture rate decreases, for example, the treatment is reported to have been a success. The difficulty with using fracture rate or clinical status as a means of judging effectiveness in any treatment of OI is extremely difficult, and often inaccurate. This is due to the large differentiation between the clinical manifestations of OI from one person to the next. Also, as many people with OI will attest, it is very common to go for months or years with no fractures, and then hit a cycle of repeated fractures for no apparent reason. Simply put, the nature of OI makes it difficult to determine what treatment modalities are conclusively beneficial.

Throughout the twentieth century, surges of interest have occurred where a stir of activity surrounds certain treatments for a period of time. As noted below in figure 12-1, from 1911 to 1981, there was considerable attention focused on vitamin D, thymus, androgens and estrogens, fluoride, and calcitonin.[3]

Figure 12-1[3]		
Years of interest	OI Treatment or Agent Studied	No. of articles
1911-1940	Vitamin D	21
1927-1943	Thymus	6
1930-1968	Androgens & estrogens	17
1966-1975	Floride	8
1972-1981	Calcitonin	16

Funding of OI Research

In the United States, biomedical research is currently and primarily funded through four sources:
- The National Institutes of Health (NIH)
- The March of Dimes Birth Defects Foundation
- Shriners Hospitals for Crippled Children
- The Osteogenesis Imperfecta Foundation, Inc.

Current OI Treatment and Research

Currently treatments to help eliminate some symptoms of OI are limited to mechanical treatments, such as intramedullary roddings, which can benefit people with OI immensely. These orthopedic procedures provide people with OI with greater functional ability through straightened and strengthened bones. In addition to these mechanical treatments, much has been learned in recent years about OI at the basic molecular level.

Genetic research is being conducted at various centers throughout the United States. This relatively new information is being made available to families and is proving to be especially beneficial to parents seeking genetic counseling. These basic molecular studies provide the basis for the hope that at some point OI could be eliminated in future generations.

So, what therapeutic treatments hold a degree of promise for people currently living with OI? It is conceivable that future therapeutic treatments could be as complex as gene therapy, or as simple as a "magic pill".

Many people with OI hope for headway in the area of gene therapy. Gene therapy is an attempt to replace the defective genes in the body. Peter Byers, M.D., Chairman of the Medical Advisory Council of the Osteogenesis Imperfecta Foundation, recently stated, "I believe that gene therapy is the least likely workable method of treatment for OI in the immediate future."[2]

Gene therapy looks very promising for cystic fibrosis and other recessively inherited disorders where there are no functional genes to begin with. In cystic fibrosis, there is hope that the defective gene can be supplemented by the addition of a single normal copy of the gene. In OI, the situation is somewhat different. People with most forms of OI have one normal copy of the gene and one altered copy that codes for an abnormal protein. Since this combination of normal and abnormal protein copies produce OI, gene therapy would have to remove just the altered copy, a very difficult task with current technology. One of the additional problems we face in OI is how to deliver the therapy so it can affect all the bones of the body. Further, people would be treated at a time when many bony alterations have already occurred so that replacement of the genes that produce the collagen proteins might not be able to alter the structure or growth of bones that are growing on an altered scaffolding. Finally, gene therapy research and treatment currently is very expensive, and is very much in the pioneer stages.

Some investigators hold promise for gene therapy, but they all agree that any advances in this area are many years in the future.

In conclusion, people with OI and their caregivers must look to continued research, clinical trials, and new developments for future advances in therapy. It is important to maintain a healthy curiosity about and interest in new reports of positive results of treatments for OI. Although there is no one agent that has been proven conclusively to benefit people with OI, it is important to continue the search for effective treatments for the causes and symptoms of OI.

Endnotes

1. **Albright, James A., MD**, *Systemic Treatment of Osteogenesis Imperfecta, Clinical Orthopaedics and Related Research*, 159:88, 1981.
2. **Griffith, J.P.C.**, *Idiopathic osteopsathyrosis (Fragilitas Ossium) in infancy and childhood, American Journal of Medical Science*, 113:426, 1897.
3. **Albright**, p. 88.
4. **Byers, Peter, MD**, *Personal interview, June 1994.*

Figure 12-2 *oim* or OI Mouse

This mouse has a defect that is similar to one found in a child with a rare recessively inherited form of OI. Mice, (or other animals with OI), provide scientists with ways to test many different forms of therapy that may, ultimately, help people who have OI.

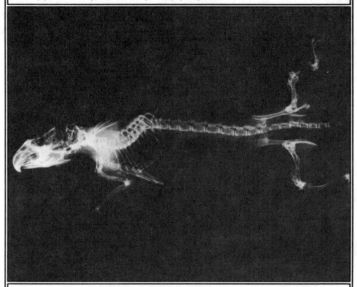

Panel A: A whole body x-ray of the *oim*/(OI murine) - a mouse with a recessively inherited form of osteogenesis imperfecta. The spine is curved, the ribs are thin, and the bones show fractures that have healed or are healing.

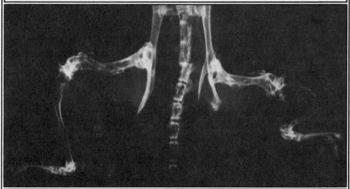

Panel B: A closeup of the femurs in *oim* showing loss of mineral and fractures.

Chapter 13

Psychology of OI within the Family

by David E. C. Cole, M.D., Ph.D.
Banting Institute, Toronto, Canada
and Brad McRae, Ed.D.
McRae and Associates

OI is a complex and diverse disorder that affects each individual and family in a unique way. The extent to which differences resulting from OI change lives depends on the severity of the disorder, its history, the extent to which it modifies physical appearance, and personal mobility and the presence of other family members who have OI. These factors may also influence the manner in which individuals with OI adjust to their community and work environment. It is important that the complex psychological and social aspects of OI be widely appreciated and understood.

The recognition and coping skills associated with these factors should help people who have OI lead fulfilling and productive lives.

Birth, Parents, and Family

The behavior and attitude of the parents of a child born with OI usually depends on several factors, one being their previous experience(s) with OI. For those to whom the birth of a child with OI is a complete surprise, immediate reactions are often tempered by the degree of visible deformity and apparent disability, but almost always a degree of initial shock is experienced. This reaction is often followed by anger, usually

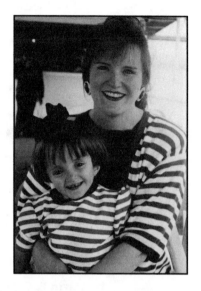

unexpressed, compounded by difficulty in locating knowledgeable personnel to explain the disorder to the parents. Feelings of guilt and subsequent depression are common as the parents learn that they may have a defective gene. It is not uncommon for parents to go through a process of mourning for the loss of the "normal" child they expected.

For the child born into a family with at least one other affected member, the psychological and social environments may be more secure. On the positive side, most families will have already adopted appropriate behavioral strategies to deal with the OI. Parents come to accept that they can prepare their affected child to deal with the medical and physical problems of OI, but they will be constantly concerned about maintaining the right environment for their child. In this situation, the parents may attempt to compensate for the loss of the "normal child" they expected by overprotecting and overindulging their own affected children.

Often when a child has a disability, the family must make considerable changes in lifestyle and become accustomed to the financial and psychological sacrifices that may become necessary. At times, members of the extended family are seen as a hindrance to the family's interaction. Grandparents, aunts, and uncles may deny the condition or even reject the child. At the other extreme, relatives may overreact and show inappropriate or undue concern for the affected child. Time and patience may modify these reactions considerably.

Initially, hospital personnel may be uncertain about how to

handle the infant. Parents generally learn the necessary skills to care for their fragile child, and then may become frustrated when medical personnel are insensitive to practical suggestions they offer. It is important that the complex psychological and social aspects of OI be widely appreciated. It is important that parents deal with their feelings as they start to cope with these difficult types of situations.

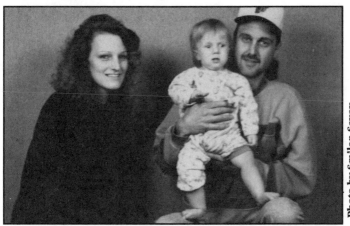

Photo by Smilen Savov

The need for parents to enjoy time away from the family either alone or together as a couple, is critical. Often parents are very afraid, or refuse to turn the care of their fragile child over to another. Fear of a fracture occurring while in the care of someone outside the family may contribute towards parents going for years before they permit themselves time away from their child with OI. Alternatively, when parents do become comfortable with the idea of obtaining respite care for their child, care becomes difficult to obtain. Parents of children with OI may experience difficulty obtaining the services of a baby-sitter, daycare, or pre-school for their child with OI.

The Delayed Diagnosis

"Our son started breaking his bones when he was a year old but OI wasn't diagnosed until he was three years old. During that time we were accused of child abuse many times. We couldn't believe that people could think that of us. My first reaction was to question whether I was somehow responsible. How could any fit mother not know why her child was always breaking bones? It was

*such a relief to finally know what was wrong with him
even though the diagnosis was a bad one."*

Children, who are less severely affected with OI, may suffer
repeated fractures before a diagnosis is made. The unexplained
fractures may raise the suspicion of child abuse in the minds of hospital
personnel, particularly when this suspicion is shared by others in the
family or community. Parents may feel extreme guilt, frustration, and
anxiety.

Growing Up

*"I learned not to ask questions about OI because I knew
the doctors didn't have the answers. My parents asked
many questions [but] they resigned themselves to just
treating the fractures as they occurred, nothing more".*

Once the diagnosis is established, most parents learn to cope.
Like all parents of children who are disabled, parents of children with
OI need an abundance of patience, courage, and faith. They may find it
difficult in some instances to persuade others of the degree of their
child's limitations, not knowing whether fractures will occur during
everyday activities. Constant awareness of their child's frailty makes
routine activities a source of crisis in everyday living. In addition,
parents may be challenged by the physical expectations society often
places on its children to participate in sports and take physical risks.

As the family begins to adapt to the condition, an imbalance may
develop if one parent becomes over-involved with the child and the
other parent and siblings take on a lesser role. As well, having an
affected child can intensify the parental desire for unaffected children.
However, this is often counterbalanced in OI families by fears of
recurrence, concerns about the need for additional special care, and
economic limitations.

Siblings

*"My brother with OI rarely has to lift a finger around the
house while the rest of us have chores to do all the time.
I often feel like his slave or his bodyguard. Although my
mom tries not to ask me to do too much because she
knows I get bitter, my other brothers and I still feel put
out. We argue over who has to put his wheelchair into
the car."*

As with adults, children also must adjust to the "loss of the dream" when a brother or sister with OI is born instead of the able-bodied sibling they had envisioned. The traits of compassion and understanding must be taught in order to avoid negative sibling relationships within the family. Parents are advised to be sensitive to feelings of:

- Jealousy - "He gets all the attention."
- Guilt - "Even though we were arguing, I didn't mean to cause the fracture."
- Bitterness - "I always have to reach things for my sister. She is such a pain."
- Inadequacy - "Because my brother has OI, it seems like my parents have higher and unfair expectations from me."
- Embarrassment - "Whenever we go anywhere, people stare."
- Pity - "I feel sorry for my brother when he has a fracture or has to go to the hospital."
- Fear of ongoing responsibilities - "It's clear that my sister will need ongoing assistance and support through the years. I dread being solely responsible for her care when my parents are no longer alive."

Parents of children with OI must take extra precautions to ensure that all their children feel loved and appreciated. It is so important that open communication exist within families who have children with OI.

It is especially, important for parents to consider the feelings of a sibling who may have been the cause of a fracture. When feelings of revenge and retaliation toward the child with OI exist, and a fracture occurs, the sibling can be racked with guilt and remorse. Siblings of children with OI should be encouraged to discuss their feelings about their

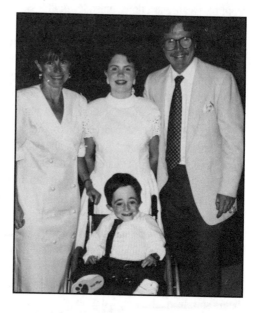

brother or sister even though those feeling may at times be negative.

A difficult situation can surface within the home when a younger sibling who does not have OI achieves mobility. Creativity becomes necessary as parents develop methods to protect the child with OI from his/her sibling. Playpens, gates, and other means of separation may become necessary until the toddler reaches an age where he/she understands the need for restrained interaction.

Going to School

"We have had a few problems since moving...to a new school - one being that he was put into a soccer team and played goalie! I just could not believe it when he told me, especially as everything had been explained in detail to the principal. [The principal] seems to think that I had exaggerated his condition and was reluctant to...make allowances for him even when he has had a fracture".

Going to school may be particularly frightening for children with OI, and for their parents, who must struggle to accept that the benefits of academic and social growth outweigh the physical risks. Children with OI will find it harder to realize these benefits if they are excluded from all activities and interactions with their peers. This could result from physical restrictions, episodes of illness, or avoidance by peers and peers' families.

Parents may also be reluctant to work with school personnel because of previous negative experiences with other "human service providers." This situation is of particular concern to parents of children affected with milder OI who appear "normal" but are at risk for fractures from a thoughtless shove by another child. Some parents feel that, if people were aware of their child's disorder, they would treat the child as "completely different," rather than different in relation to the risk of fracturing. Teachers and other school personnel, lacking accurate information, may also place inappropriate and unnecessary restrictions on the child with OI.

Children with OI have normal intelligence, yet these children may underachieve and may sometimes do worse academically than their healthy peers. Chronic illness and physical disability create special problems that hinder performance in school. All such children should receive an educational program to address these concerns, rather than being simplistically regarded as experiencing "behavioral or motivational problems."

Adolescence

Older children who are severely affected can become concerned about problems associated with inaccessibility when wheelchair use is

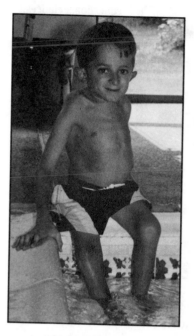

necessary. Also social problems associated with short stature and deformities sometimes become troublesome. There are many different social strategies that can be used to promote appropriate adaptation to disabling conditions like OI. Those that are self-limiting, such as withdrawal and concealment tend to promote the loss of self-esteem. Productive coping strategies include increased assertiveness in which the individual becomes more socially active and insist that more positive or neutral values be attributed to OI itself within the context of their social interactions.

During adolescence, concerns about physical appearance, sexual development, and peer acceptance are heightened. Depression and feelings of inadequacy may be problematic during this often troublesome time of life. It is therefore understandable that many parents of adolescents with OI become concerned again about the future of their children.

It is often difficult for parents to think of "letting go" of a child who has always needed their help and support. Adolescents will therefore benefit from thoughtful and careful counseling about the sometimes extra-difficult entry into adulthood and independence.

Adulthood

For the individual who is severely affected by OI, the problems of immobility and of social and financial dependence often become most troublesome in young adulthood. Affected adults may be dependant on family, friends, and neighbors for mobility. At the same time, many potential helpers are deterred from assisting those in greatest need by the fear they will be responsible for new fractures. Less than ideal accessibility may contribute to physical and social isolation and restrict

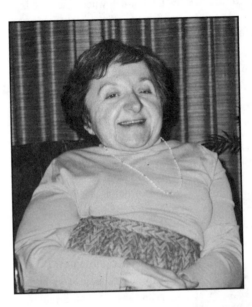

occupational and educational choices. Discrimination in the work place is sometimes prevalent, and fair financial compensation for work done is not always received. In summary, the real problems arising from the physically disabling aspects of OI, hindrances perceived by employers, acquaintances, and potential relations with the opposite sex, place great barriers between the adult with OI and his/her life goals. As adults they face the likelihood of new fractures and hospital stays. In a busy and aggressive society, they must compete on an equal basis with their physically healthy counterparts but may experience difficulty in obtaining health insurance or receiving dispensation for legitimate absences from work.

People with milder forms of OI have unique problems arising from the conflict between their outwardly normal appearance and their underlying fragility. "Who do I tell about my condition? Will it help me or hinder me to explain my absences from work related to OI by explaining the nature of the condition? When do I tell my date or my steady?" These questions are increasingly faced by adults with OI in today's world.

OI and the Health Care Professions

"Our daughter was diagnosed as having OI [type III] following a serious fracture that occurred when she was a year and a half old. After accusing us of child abuse, the doctor treated the fracture and proceeded to send

her home. We knew that there was something wrong with her because every time we would pick her up, she would scream with pain. We demanded that some tests be done. After doing the tests, they diagnosed her as having OI. The doctors offered my husband and me no hope of treatment, telling us that there was nothing that could be done, but that she could live her life in a glass cage. For a long time after that, all we could do was a lot of crying".

When first confronted with a newborn or young child with multiple fractures with or without deformities, many inexperienced health care professionals feel lost. Medical literature is limited and virtually no training exists for dealing with the kinds of problems that parents of children with OI get to know only too well. Therefore, it is important to consider several important principles when choosing medical professionals to care for the child with OI.

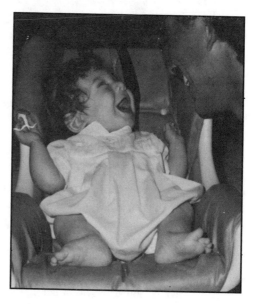

First, look for those health care professionals interested in treating the whole patient. For the medical specialist, this means referral to other specialists, or participation in treatment teams with para-medical professionals that can help with the evaluation and treatment of all the aspects of OI. Nurses and allied personnel who are likely to deal more intimately with these patients during hospital admissions should familiarize themselves with the patient's current level of activity, and thus schedule daily activities appropriately. They should not avoid handling the infant or child for fear of fractures or insist that the child participate in activities that might precipitate fractures.

Second, look for medical professionals that can refer new families to those familiar with the condition through an OI clinic, another family with a similarly affected child, or the National Brittle Bone Foundation. Although some families initially reject these overtures, they may respond later recognizing that talking with other families who have experience with raising a child with OI is extremely helpful.

Third, health care personnel should be able to listen to the parents. Parents, especially more experienced ones, will know their child's capabilities better than anyone else.

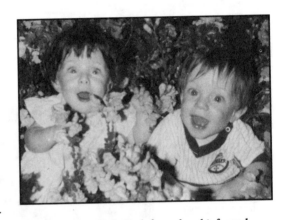

Fourth, medical professionals need to be prepared to offer psychological and social support when it is needed. Both formal and informal counseling may make a substantial difference to individuals who are dealing with the anger, grief, guilt, anxiety, and depression that OI can bring. Because OI is an uncommon, complex, and serious disorder, its presence can place considerable demand on the family, community, and society. Progressive deformities are among the most debilitating prospects for people with OI who are severely affected and for their families. A communal effort and mutual support are both needed to ensure that each person attains his or her maximum potential for personal growth. Developing a better response to the psychological and social issues will help to balance the current scientific efforts to expand the understanding of the genetic defects and their psychological consequences.

Works Cited

Cole, D.E.C., *Psychosocial Aspects of Osteogenesis Imperfecta: An Update, American Journal of Medical Genetics*, 45:207-211, 1993. *Permission donated by John Wiley & Sons, Inc.*

Shea-Landry, G.L., Cole, D.E.C., *Psychosocial Aspects of Osteogenesis Imperfecta, Canadian Medical Journal*, 135:977-981, 1986.

Chapter 14

Key Elements in Developing Self-esteem

By Sandra Pinkerton, Ed.D.
Fort Lee, New Jersey

Issues of self-esteem appear in the forefront of daily life. Self-esteem is the belief we have in ourselves and the self-respect that accompanies that belief. Although the issues are numerous, there are several key factors identified for a high self-esteem. A person's self-esteem can fluctuate during crisis periods, ill-health, life-style changes, and with relationships with family, friends, peers and/or co-workers.

Recently, while the Winter Olympics were being shown on television, a segment about a young female figure skater from Canada was highlighted. The skater revealed she had taken a self-concept inventory and scored very low in the area of self-esteem. My first reaction to this disclosure was one of amazement. How could a woman who qualifies in skating for the Olympics not feel good about herself? How could a person with a body of grace and strength feel so poorly about her abilities and capabilities?

Upon further reflection, my thoughts turned to how people with OI, like myself, can have a positive self-image when we encounter roadblocks that are accentuated by physical and/or sensory impairments. Coping with OI can be an overwhelming task. The architectural, communication, and personal barriers we experience on a daily basis are a constant challenge to sustaining our self-esteem.

Clemes and Bean[1] summarized years of research and assessed four basic conditions necessary for high self-esteem. These conditions are:

- A sense of connectiveness
- A sense of uniqueness
- A sense of power
- A sense of models

Connectiveness

Although all of the above conditions are important to the self-esteem of people with OI, connecting with the people around us is the foundation upon which self-esteem develops. We first learn self-esteem from the comments made to or about us as we develop. These comments come from our parent(s), siblings, playmates, friends, teachers, and later, workmates.

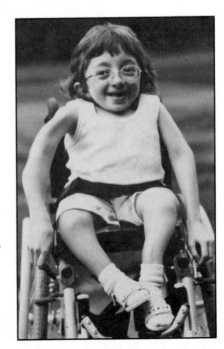

As children with OI, we have little control over parents', siblings' or teachers' fears of our well-being and their overprotectiveness. It is a natural reaction of those who are responsible for our care. We cannot blame family members for being overprotective since throughout history, persons with disabilities have been portrayed as dependent. Taking charge of our relationships with family members, at whatever age we are able to do so, can provide us with the framework to feel that we belong in a positive manner. Once we establish a sense of belonging as an integral member within our families, it is important to reach beyond them to schoolmates, friends, or coworkers.

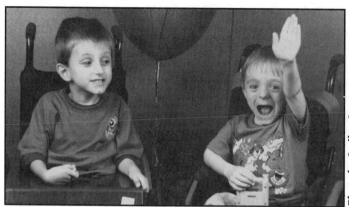

Photo by Smilen Savov

In order for extended connections to occur, we have to be worth connecting to. Our interests and skills can foster this connection to others. If we are unable to physically leave home because of health or lack of transportation, we should consider inviting people to visit us. Learning to play games, cards, or other hobbies that can be undertaken at home provides enjoyment and the chance to be with others. Another possibility is to review a video and invite friends over to see it. Sports events are enjoyable to view with others, and the television offers plenty of them from which to choose. Hobby or craft clubs could also meet at your home, and would provide further contacts outside of the immediate family.

Friendship is a component of connectiveness. It is as vital to our well-being as happiness. Good friends are hard to make and even harder to keep. According to The New York Times article on "Maintaining Friendships for the Sake of Your Health,"[2] friends can fill a variety of roles, and no one friend should be expected to satisfy them all. Friends can join us in pursuing pleasurable recreational activities, they can provide intellectual stimulation, and they can enhance the joys of personal celebrations.

Most importantly, friends can help to reaffirm our self-worth, even when circumstances beyond our control challenge our sense of competence and self-esteem. Establishing close friendships does involve risk taking, but the risks far outweigh the feelings of loneliness associated with not having a friend. A close friend shares the good and bad times, and sometimes is the one who is supportive when our self-esteem is low. This close friend may come to us through many avenues, but most often for people with OI, it is necessary for us to reach out to others and try to help them feel comfortable around us. This may seem unfair, but the unfairness compounds if we are left without a friend because we did not make the extra effort to reach out.

Depending upon individual circumstances, a person can begin to make every attempt to connect with others by joining community and/or professional groups, civic or religious organizations. These groups have specific goals and offer many opportunities for socialization which may lead to relationships outside the group or organizational activities.

Uniqueness

Unfortunately, we live in a society that values conformity. In some ways, by the nature of our disabilities we are not expected to be "like

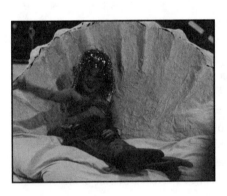

other people", and yet are expected at the same time to conform to standards we are unable to meet or maintain. For example, as a teenager I wanted to be part of a group - wear the same clothes, think the same thoughts, and view life as the group saw it. Later, I realized that I did not fit into this group no

matter how hard I tried. I could not wear the same clothes because of size, bracing, and ease of dressing. I did not think the same thoughts because I did not have the same awareness level and I could not view life in the same way because of my unique experiences. As I reached that realization, and in a sense matured, I concentrated on me and began to accomplish tasks and express myself in my own way. This was much easier once I passed adolescence.

Uniqueness is what makes us who we are. It means acknowledging and respecting qualities that make us different. This acknowledge-

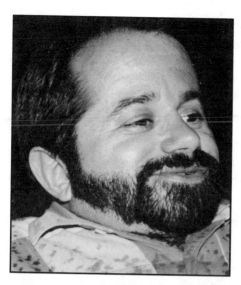

ment and respect attributed to ourselves will help others to admire us for possessing these qualities. Our outward demeanor of a high self-esteem will make it more difficult for people to "feel sorry for us." (Most of us cannot tolerate pity!)

Power

Power lies within all of us. Each of us has the ability to feel powerful. This feeling of power comes from knowing that we have the capability and opportunity to influence the circumstances of our own lives. At times, it appears that we have no control of our lives, but the control of our destiny is within us. The stresses of prejudice and discrimination can be minimized if we are able to truly convince ourselves that we have the power to cope with our daily frustrations.

Taking responsibility for our behavior is a component of power. If we have failed at a task, we should not be afraid to try it again and again. We need to try to avoid feeling defeated to such a degree that we start blaming others for our failures. There are times when other people are at fault, but looking at our contribution to the situation or interaction is a good way to begin to understand the reasons for our behavior and the behavior of the others.

Another component of power is decision-making. When we were young, other people made decisions for us. As we mature, we should take on greater responsibilities and begin making decisions ourselves. If we are not prepared to independently make decisions, we may need to seek help from others. Generally, most decisions do not have to be made immediately. Consulting other people, reviewing alternatives, asking questions of friends, family, and professionals whom we respect, can prove helpful in arriving at a decision. No matter what input we obtain, the final decision lies within us. In fact, it is important to remember the consequences of our decisions are generally not life threatening or irreparable.

Taking risks gives us a sense of power also. Risk-taking is perhaps one of the most difficult things to do and it is vital for our future happiness. We usually will have no idea where the risk may take us, but if we fail to try, we will never know the excitement and fulfillment that can come from extending beyond ourselves. Then we are able to learn about our inner strength, and the sense of power that comes from possessing that strength.

None of life's endeavors can begin without respecting ourselves and others. No matter how many times we have been hurt, rejected, or made to feel "different" because of OI, we must repeat to ourselves "I am a worthwhile human being. I have strengths and weaknesses. I have the right to self-fulfillment." OI cannot be allowed to rule our lives. It is only one aspect of who we are and our uniqueness.

Role Models

Recent legislation has emphasized that people with disabilities must be included in all aspects of community living. This inclusion should help raise our self-esteem. However, we may be in a position where we may not necessarily have someone with the same disability or others with disabilities as role models. Although role models do not have to look or think in the same way, they should assist us to establish meaningful values, goals, ideals, and standards.

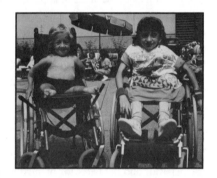

If at all possible, people with OI must connect with others with OI. Discovering how others with the same disability cope with daily frustrations is better medicine than a doctor could prescribe. Laughing and crying together is healthier than laughing and crying alone.

By organizing support groups, either through face-to-face meetings, letters, or newsletters, we can increase our awareness of others with disabilities, and speak out about our needs and rights as fully participating citizens. The establishment of this bond can be strengthened by organizing or joining support groups.

We want to be consulted. We want to contribute to the betterment of society and ourselves. We want others to realize that with the experience of having OI, we are the experts about attitudinal, communication, and architectural barriers.

These groups can encourage the development of a positive self-image and self-esteem. Others with OI can promote a sense of power and the development and reinforcement of our identity. They can help us to understand that our limitations can be artificial, as well as real. They can provide us with role models or encourage us to become the models.

The future lies in our brains and how we view ourselves. It lies in our ability to connect with the world around us. It lies in the unique qualities we now have and will develop. It lies in how we use the power we possess and how we present that sense of power as a role model to others.

Endnotes

1. **Clemes, H., Bean, R.**, *Self Esteem: The Key to Your Child's Well Being, Putnam's Sons, New York, 1981.*
2. *"Maintaining Friendships for the Sake of Your Health," New York Times, February, 1993.*

Chapter 15

Dating, Intimacy, and Your Child with OI

by Beth Tatman
Maitland, Florida

I believe that a child, no matter how severely affected by OI, can become a happy, loving, and sexual adult. Parents, please know that you are not alone in your desire to seek answers and solutions to the challenges your child will face in life. Inside I feel very much like my sisters, but my outward appearances remind me that in other ways I am not like them at all. Like many others with OI, I have an elongated lower jaw, pigeon chest, multiple scars from surgeries, and am short-statured. I use a wheelchair for mobility.

The most important attribute which qualifies me to address the delicate subject of sexual intimacy is that I am a happy, loving, and sexual adult with OI. A teenager with OI once called me "the proof of the pudding."

Like many others with OI, I was the only person in my family to have this condition. I did not meet anyone else with OI until I was 25 years old. By then I had a good job, a car, an apartment, and a well-established social life, just like many other motivated, self-confident single women of the day. Of course, there were many differences between me and other women.

My 70 major fractures and 17 orthopaedic surgeries tell me that many of my experiences have made my life somewhat different from others my age.

In 1985 I married Jim Tatman, a wonderful man who was an attorney. Our very happy, rewarding marriage ended in June 1990 with his untimely death from complications of surgery. My interest in the subject of intimacy for people with disabilities began after a 21-year-old friend told me her story. She is very small and severely affected by OI. She was in college and had met a man she found interesting. He seemed interested in her also. She scheduled her first gynecological exam and Pap test and requested oral contraceptives. The physician, who had never had a patient like her, refused to conduct the exam and told her she could never have sex. She was very discouraged, and I was furious with the doctor for being so narrow-minded in his views on sexuality and for his unwillingness to conduct a gynecological exam in other than the traditional "feet-in-the-stirrups" fashion. Fortunately for my friend, she didn't follow his advise. Even though she is not able to engage in intercourse, she and her partner today share a very mutually satisfying sex life.

In order to help my friend, and many others like her, I began a formal quest for information. I attended a series of workshops on human sexuality with the goal of developing some expertise on the intimacy and sexuality concerns commonly faced by people with OI. In short, I learned that few "experts" could provide any meaningful counsel for people with disabilities, and of course, no one knew a thing about the unique concerns of people with OI. After repeatedly receiving unsatisfactory answers to my questions and concerns, I reached my limit of endurance and began to voice my frustration. When I was encouraged to conduct a sexuality workshop myself, I jumped at the opportunity.

I began conducting intimacy, dating, and sexuality workshops for the Osteogenesis Imperfecta Foundation, at their 1984 national conference. The workshop was designed only for adults with OI and their "significant others"; non-affected parents or medical professionals were not invited to attend. This was to ensure that participants would feel comfortable to open up and truly share their concerns and, believe me, this was an open group!

Prior to this first gathering, I distributed a questionnaire to many adults with OI who were willing to volunteer information concerning their sexuality. The participants had the option to remain anonymous. Most provided very in-depth answers. While the results were very interesting, they were not surprising to me. All the participants desired social and sexual interaction, but few of their parents had ever discussed even the basics of sexuality or implied in any way that they thought their children would be sexually active as adults. Their physicians had also failed to bring up the subject of sexuality, and few were able to enter into an informed discussion after the subject was brought up. The majority of the respondents had received their sexual knowledge from friends and siblings, but few were dealing with the real issues faced by persons with OI. Among the survey group, which ranged in age from the late teens to the mid-70's, approximately 75 percent of the women and 50 percent of the men had no sexual experience.

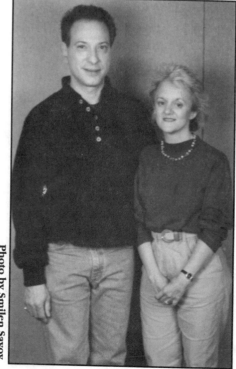

Photo by Smilen Savov

Lack of physical contact was another area of concern that was expressed repeatedly; some had been hugged very seldom and never kissed. The problem cited foremost was finding someone with whom to interact. It was not unusual for their partners to be concerned about physically hurting the partner with OI.

I continued my pursuit of issues of intimacy and sexu-ality for several important reasons.

First of all, no one was talking to people with OI about sex, and there were many unanswered questions. Secondly, there was no literature available that met their specific needs. Most people with OI had no role models to demonstrate that a healthy sexual relationship could be achieved. Thirdly, and most importantly, some people had received erroneous information about sexuality from well-respected medical professionals. It was important to me that the myths and incorrect information had to be dismissed.

Since that first workshop in 1984, I have conducted intimacy workshops at the majority of the Foundation conferences. The 1992 conference included separate workshops for affected adults, for teens with OI and their unaffected siblings, and for parents and medical professionals. In my workshops I take an "open forum" approach, in which the participants determine the issues to be discussed. Often, the participants, especially the adults, learn the most simply by sharing concerns and experiences with each other.

Now let me share with you some of the valuable concepts that have been shared at these workshops.

Parental Influence

As a parent, you are the one with the greatest influence over your child's development. You can provide adequate medical care and a good education. You can foster in your children high self-esteem, self-confidence, worthwhile values, a sense of humor, a spirit of adventure, and good problem-solving skills. But, just as importantly, family life is where we first start to develop healthy relationships and intimacy with others.

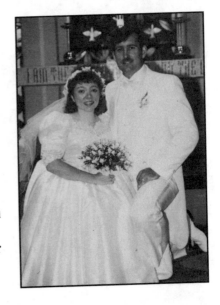

You have been given a very fragile human being to love, shelter, teach, and mold into a happy, productive adult member of society. When you look at your child, can you imagine him or her head over heels in love, sexually active, married, or as a parent? It is often difficult for any parent to think about these situations when the child is very young, especially when the child has special needs.

Need for Intimacy of People with OI

Your child will grow up to have the same hopes, dreams, and desires as any other adult, as well as the same emotional and physical needs. Persons with OI have the same need and capacity for intimacy as anyone else. Why single out this necessary subject for discussion? Because your child with OI will be socialized differently and will most likely have to face additional issues and areas of concern that you, your other children, and his peers will never face.

Social Experiences

Remember when you had your first platonic "girlfriend" or "boyfriend?" Family members probably asked you, "Is she pretty?" or, "Is he cute?" Very few people asked if he or she was smart or well-behaved. Appearance was the most important characteristic called to our attention at that very early age.

Later, when you were a teenager, your thoughts and feelings about members of the opposite sex changed. Your experiences turned to boy/girl dances, dating, going steady, or the old arm around the shoulders that slips a little lower in the darkness of a movie theater.

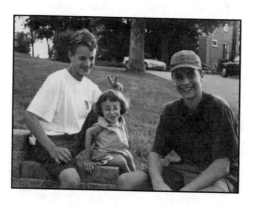

This possibly becomes the time of the first date, the first kiss, the first serious relationship, or the first experience with sexual intercourse. At the same time, you learned how to dress and act by associating with others your age. All of this was part of your social and sexual learning process. You were receiving very subtle messages from the people around you. You were learning what behavior was acceptable.

Unfortunately, your child with OI may not have the same experiences. Crutches, braces, casts, and wheelchairs can make it difficult to dance or hold hands. Your child may not obtain a driver's license as soon as others, because of the lack of adaptive equipment or driver training programs. Dating is difficult today without a car. Added physical barriers such as inaccessible friends' homes, normal teenage hangouts like malls or movie theaters, or special school events held in inaccessible places may force your child to stay home. At the same time, your child will probably become known by most everyone at school and in your community. This "celebrity" status can shine an almost unbearable spotlight on a young person trying to make friends, pursuing a romance, or doing other things healthy teenagers do. It is also hard to get out from under watchful eyes when you have a condition like OI. Being dependent on others so often obstructs the desire to be alone with members of the opposite sex.

To many adults with OI, adolescence was the worst and most difficult time of their lives. Up to then, most had been popular with their peers. But, as boys and girls began pairing off, they wound up feeling excluded. Thankfully, the social lives of most persons with OI improve during and following the college years as they build self-esteem and develop social skills.

Physical Characteristics of OI

The physical characteristics of OI can, and often do, have a significant effect on sexuality. Some women with OI have small and/or deformed pelvic bones which can make intercourse painful or even impossible. Several women have undergone experimental surgery in an attempt to correct this problem. However, most simply learn to develop a satisfying sexual relationship by experimenting with various forms of sexual expression both they and their partners enjoy. Other common physical characteristics, such as hip contractures and "pigeon chest," can cause difficulties with positioning for intercourse. Such problems can usually be worked out with patience and experimentation.

Some people with OI may be of short stature, have bone deformities or many scars from previous surgeries, which can contribute to difficulty in feeling positive about one's self-image. The goals of parents of children with OI should be to help them to become self-confident, and learn to focus beyond their physical appearance.

Most people with OI are capable of producing offspring. Ultimately, the decision to have children lies with the person with OI and his or her partner.

Appearance is Important

Developing a fashion sense, including clothing and make-up, become important social skills. "Looks aren't everything," of course, but most kids, especially teenagers, want to dress like their peers. Many fashionable clothes are produced in smaller sizes these days, but some clothes will need to be altered. It is very important to avoid dressing your child with OI in "cute" clothes that are too childlike for his or her age simply because they fit well.

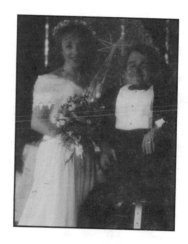

Relationships

Many people with OI will marry. Partners can be others with OI, (which is rare), people of short stature, (which is also rare), people with another type of disability, or someone who does not have any type of disability.

All people need love and support through periods when they are establishing intimate relationships. After all, the relationships we develop in this life constitute a very important, aspect of living. Parents can help by actively listening to their child's trials, frustrations, successes, and failures. Openly discussing potentially difficult situations helps children to be prepared, fortified, and confident about relationships that may develop.

Parent to Child Communication about Sexuality

You might find it difficult to talk to your child about sex and relationships. Some parents base their counsel upon deeply based religious values. Whatever your values, please do not make the mistake of treating

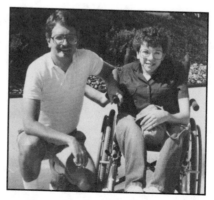

your child's sexual development as a non-issue. Many adults with OI have lamented the lack of positive reinforcement from their families on issues of dating, marriage, and having children. Several found themselves expecting babies because they thought they could not get pregnant. After a workshop, a 52-year-old man thanked me for what he had learned. All his life, he said, he had been treated like a block of wood. Now he had hope that he too could find someone. Another man had confined himself to same-sex relationships, he said, because it was easier and had thought this his only option. One woman had been told by her doctor that she could not possibly have a child like herself because there was no history of OI in her family. Her baby boy has severe OI.

Make sure your child is knowledgeable about the physical and emotional benefits of abstinence prior to marriage, about establishing a lasting relationship, about birth control and safer sex. They need to know the facts about sexually transmitted diseases and AIDS. Females need to have regular gynecological and breast examinations as well as Pap tests. Males should learn about testicular and prostate exams. Everyone needs to learn how to take responsibility for themselves and for their partners.

Conclusion

Society's perceptions of persons with all types of disabilities are changing. Hopefully, as the years pass, the ability of adults with OI to enter into healthy, loving, and mutually satisfying relationships will continue to improve. After all, if we all keep talking to each other, we will discover "the proof of the pudding" and become the successful adult role models with OI from whom we all can learn.

Chapter 16

Education of Children and Youth with OI

By Shannon R. Smith
Pittsburgh, Pennsylvania

Philosophy of Inclusive Education

Historically, many students with OI have been educated in segregated environments. The more severe their OI, the more extreme the segregation. Many times this segregation entailed being sent to another school district or to another school within their own district. Even those who were fortunate enough to attend their neighborhood schools often spent at least part, if not all, of the day segregated from their non-disabled peers.

Fortunately, this is changing as more children with OI now attend their neighborhood schools in regular classrooms. This type of educational programming is called inclusive education. Inclusive education means that ALL students attend their neighborhood schools with their same age peers, and are provided with the supports necessary to fully benefit from their educational experiences.

Parents of children with OI need to be aware of their child's right to receive a full education in "the least restrictive environment." The least restrictive environment would entitle most children with OI to be educated in a regular classroom environment where they can benefit from the stimulation and social contact, and where appropriate supportive supplementary assistance is provided when necessary. This is often referred to as "mainstreaming."

Where do I begin?

Begin by asking questions and developing a better understanding of the Individuals with Disabilities Education Act (IDEA), Public Law 102-119. IDEA, formerly the Education for the Handicapped Act (EHA), is a federal law that supports special education and related service programming and guarantees a free appropriate public education to children with disabilities. It is also important that parents familiarize themselves with similar laws, some of which have been amended periodically, including the Education of All Handicapped Children Act (EAHCA) or Public Law 94-142.

In order to successfully accommodate all children within the

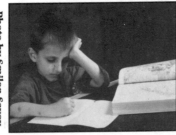

school system, school census takers should ask if there is a child with a handicapping condition in the household. However, whether information is obtained by the school or not, parents should inform their local school district about possible future needs at the time of diagnosis of OI. This information will allow the school sufficient time to budget for any needed services and will, hopefully, forestall any delay in provisions.

Regardless of whether a child is entering the public school system at kindergarten, is transferring from a special school or from home tutoring, the approach in terms of attitude is basically the same, i.e., approach the school with a positive, cooperative and pleasant attitude.

What are the Purposes of the IDEA?

The major purposes of the IDEA are to:
- Ensure that all children with disabilities have available to them a

"free appropriate public education" that includes special education and related services designed to meet their unique needs. This applies to the full range of academic program options (such as art, music, industrial arts, consumer and homemaking education, and vocational eduation), non-academic services, physical education and extracurricular activities.

- Ensure that the rights of children and youths with disabilities and their parents are protected.
- Assist states and localities in providing for the education of all children and youth with disabilities age birth through twenty-one.
- Educate children with disabilities.

Services for Very Young Children

Services to very young children with disabilities are also covered under the IDEA. Through it, states must provide special education and related services to eligible preschool children, ages 3 through 5. Part H says that states may make services available to eligible infants and toddlers (birth through 2 years). Services for these young children are provided in different ways than are services for school-aged children. Children attending pre-school may qualify for physical or speech therapy. Some school districts may provide transportation to preschool programs, pay tuition, or provide a paraprofessional (aide) for additional staffing.

Attending day care or nursery school is a very valuable experience for a child with OI. It helps develop self-confidence, teaches them to trust adults other than their parents, and provides them with the opportunity for social contact with other children. Often, early childhood programs at special education schools are designed for the mentally or emotionally handicapped children. A community supported or church-run program may be more willing to accept children with special needs. When a child is ready for kindergarten, it helps to be able to explain that he/she had already attended a day care or nursery school program successfully.

Evaluation

The term "evaluation" refers to the process of gathering and using information to determine whether a child has a disability and the nature and extent of the special education and related services that the child will need. The public schools are required to conduct this evaluation for children at no cost to the family.

Tests are an important part of an evaluation, but the family's input is also important. Additionally, the evaluation process should include observations by professionals who have worked with the child, the child's medical history, (when it is relevant to his or her performance in school,) information and observations from the family about the child's school experiences, abilities,

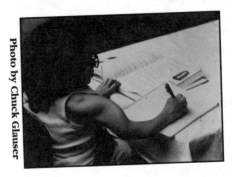

Photo by Chuck Glauser

needs, behavior outside of school, and his or her feelings about school.

The multidisciplinary team conducting the evaluation may include the following professionals, as appropriate: school psychologist, speech and language pathologist, occupational therapist, physical therapist and/or physical education therapist, medical specialists, educational diagnosticians, classroom teachers, and others.

Professionals will observe your child and may administer tests that examine your child's personality and adaptive behavior patterns, academic achievement, potential or aptitude (intelligence), functioning levels, perceptual ability, and vocational interest and aptitude. The tests must be given in a way that does not discriminate on the basis of disability or racial/cultural background.

Individualized Education Program (IEP)

An Individualized Education Program (IEP) is a written statement of the educational program designed to meet a child's, ages 3 - 21, special needs.

The IEP serves two purposes: (1) to establish the learning goals for the child and (2) to state the services that the school district will provide. The IDEA requires that every child receiving special education services have an IEP, that parents be included

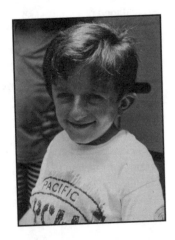

in the development of this IEP, and that the child's parents are entitled to receive their own copy of the IEP in order to keep track of progress and to maintain home records. The IEP describes the education program for your child for one school year and should be reviewed and revised every year.

A child's IEP should include statements of the child's strengths and weaknesses and should describe the instructional program developed specifically for him or her. This plan shows the child's current educational level, short and long term goals, and any special means or needs to achieve these goals. It also includes transportation and any related services your child will require. Accessible transportation, physical therapy, occupational therapy, adapted physical education, and the services of a "mobility facilitator" or "aide" are generally included for children with OI. It is very important for parents to be entirely satisfied with the IEP prior to signing it as this document will direct the services the child will receive.

• *Transportation*

Transportation services are provided to those students who need special assistance because of their disability or the location of the school relative to their home. Some students are able to use the same transportation that students without disabilities use to get to school and others require specialized transportation such as a wheelchair lift. The school district must provide travel to and from school, between schools, provide travel in and around school buildings, and provide specialized equipment, such as adapted buses, lifts, and ramps.

• *Physical Therapy*

Physical therapists are primarily concerned with developing and enhancing the physical potential of students with disabilities so that they can achieve maximum independence and function in all their educational activities. Physical therapists provide treatment to increase muscle strength, mobility, and endurance. They help to improve the student's posture, gait, and body awareness and monitor the function, fit, and proper use of mobility aids and devices. Children with OI who wear braces and benefit from daily periods of weight bearing can stand within the classroom with the use of a standing table.

• *Occupational Therapy*

Occupational therapy is provided by therapists who concentrate upon assessing and treating children with disabilities that impair their daily life functioning. By focusing upon the skills of daily living, occupational therapists can often help individual students to function in the least restrictive environment. They help to develop school and work skills in addition to play and leisure skills. Occupational therapists provide treatment to strengthen and develop fine motor functions and improve the student's ability to perform tasks necessary for independent functioning.

• *Mobility Facilitator or Aide*

Some children with OI require the services of an assistant to accomplish certain tasks within the school. An aide can help a child with OI with toileting, reaching high objects, assistance with doors and ramps, putting on and taking off braces and general safety precautions. Although sometimes difficult, it is usually better for the child if the aide remains as detached from the child as possible, i.e., serves as classroom resource rather than the child's resource. An unhealthy dependency and overcompensation can occur if precautions are not established from the start. As a child gets a little older, other classmates can often be enlisted to assist as needed, and ideally the assistance should be eliminated if possible.

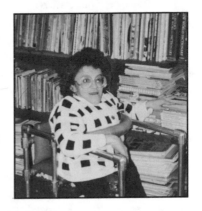

• *Accessibility and Physical Accommodations*

For a child with OI, some specific accommodations are sometimes needed at the school. A school with many steps can often be made architecturally accessible for a student who uses a wheelchair at relatively little cost by the addition of ramps and other minor modifications such as the relocation of classes. Arrangements can be made for an ambulatory child with OI to change classes a few minutes before the bell rings to help prevent unnecessary physical contact in crowded halls. If the family has special equipment for accomplishing some necessary activity, it may help to offer this equipment for school use. A separate set of books can be kept at home for the student's use to avoid the need to carry heavy books for homework. A urinary bottle can be kept in the bathroom for the use of a boy in a wheelchair.

- ### *Recess and Adapted Physical Education*

For many children with OI, the recess and physical education periods are most challenging. To accommodate children who wish to play without the threat of physical harm, a "protected play area" within the regular playground is ideal. Constructed with barriers to prevent balls and other safety hazards from harming the children, a protected play area can house tables, safe play equipment, and resemble a gazebo.

As physical education is provided for all children, adapted physical education is appropriate for many children with OI. Many sports, physical skills, and recreational pursuits can be learned by children with OI, which often provide much enjoyment throughout life. The structure of the adapted physical education class depends greatly upon the needs of those enrolled, the creativity of the teacher, and the details discussed in the IEP.

- ### *Private Tutoring*

For many children with OI, it occasionally becomes necessary to receive instruction in the hospital or at home. This is often required following surgery, or when long periods of immobilization are in order following a fracture. To eliminate excessive absences and missed assignments, a tutor can work individually with the child. Generally, the tutor obtains textbooks and class assignments from the teacher, and instructs a designated number of hours per week in the child's home.

How to Get Services Increased

Suppose your child gets physical therapy once per month, and you think he or she needs therapy weekly. What do you do? First, you can talk with your child's therapist and school principal and request an IEP review meeting with the purpose of increasing physical therapy services. Discuss the child's needs and review evaluations of his or her progress. The school personnel will either agree with you and change the IEP, or they will disagree with you. With any disagreement, you can appeal the decision of the IEP team. You may need to seek advice from the Parent Information and Training Project in your state. Your local department of special education can provide you with your state's guidelines for providing services in your state and for appealing decisions.

What about College?

In most cases, the only deterrent facing the student with OI in

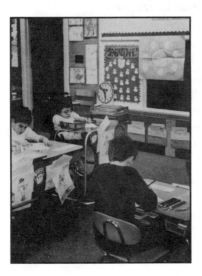

choosing a college with optimum accessibility of both the learning and living facilities. Many colleges and universities have support services to assist in the accommodation of students with disabilities. Personnel providing these services can often be helpful in providing information to help prospective students determine whether or not the college will meet their needs. A visit to any considered college is imperative in order to judge the degree of accessibility.

Conclusion

It is helpful to understand the valuable experience of one individual with OI in mainstream education. The following quote from Doug Lathrop, an adult with OI from California, says it well:

"Sometimes when people ask me if I look back fondly on my experience as a mainstreamed student, I tell them about a reunion I attended during my senior year in high school. It was a reunion of my class from the elementary school for disabled children that I attended from kindergarten through sixth grade. All who attended there had some form of disability. A few of us had been mainstreamed along the way, but most had continued in the segregated school for students with disabilities.

I especially looked forward to seeing my closest friends, the two classmates who had attended regular junior high and high schools as I had. For the three of us, the event was a sobering experience. First, we were the only ones who had driven to the reunion. We were the only ones, in fact, who knew how to drive. My two friends and I were full of stories about what we had done since elementary school and were eager to talk about our plans for college and the careers we wanted to pursue. The others had not done much since I had seen them last, and their futures did not look too bright either. Their pained, longing looks seemed to indicate a fear of physical harm if they so much as opened their mouths.

I can't say junior high is something I remember fondly. It was painful, it was traumatic. For a long time, those were years I wanted to forget. But after seeing the world of fear and dependency into which so many of my old friends had retreated, I became grateful for the opportunity I got to escape the same fate an opportunity they never had. If given a chance to change things, I would have had chosen a main-streamed learning environment much sooner- kindergarten, perhaps."

Works Cited

National Information Center for Children and Youth with Disabiliites, Questions often Asked About Special Education Services, Washington, DC, 1993.

Osteogenesis Imperfecta Foundation, Inc., The Education of a Child with Osteogenesis Imperfecta, Tampa, FL, 1989.

Chapter 17

Child Abuse Accusations - A Fragile Issue

by Heidi C. Glauser, Pittsburgh, Pennsylvania
Rosalind James, Long Island, New York
and Douglas Lathrop, Northridge, California

Picture this - a young mother carries her crying two-year-old daughter into the emergency room. "She just tripped on the doormat and now something is wrong with her right leg," she states. Suspecting a fractured tibia, a full series of X-rays are taken. The recent tibia fracture is visible as are fractures of the ribs, clavicle and left humerus, all in various stages of healing. The first thought that entered the attending physician's mind was, "Could this possibly be child abuse?"

At this point, the course of events can take one of two tracks. Either the films and symptoms are reviewed more intensely, and osteogenesis imperfecta, or brittle bones, is diagnosed, or the family enters into a nightmarish ordeal involving false accusations, misdiagnosis, and trauma to all concerned.

"Child abuse is a major problem," said Peter Byers, M.D., chairman of the Osteogenesis Imperfecta Foundation Medical Advisory Committee. "We've become very sensitized to child abuse without a commensurate sensitivity to OI. Osteogenesis Imperfecta is a rare condition, which affects one in 25,000 people. Child abuse is far more common. So, if you're looking at something common, a relatively rare cause can slip by."[1]

Over the past decade, American society as a whole has stepped up its efforts to protect its children from abuse. In many ways, this increased vigilance is welcome. It follows a period of silence on the subject, a time when many abused children were left unprotected by schools, physicians, social-service agencies, family members, and others in a position to help them. Child abuse is a behavioral disease, a pattern of behavior that often is passed down from one generation to the next. Many abusive parents were themselves abused as children. Open, honest discussion of the issue not only can ensure the safety of countless children but can encourage parents who wish to break the cycle of abusive behavior to seek the help they need in doing so.

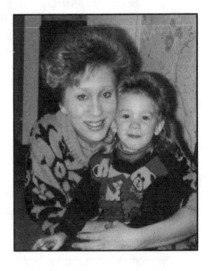

This newfound awareness, unfortunately, has not been accompanied by greater public awareness of OI. Most of the false child abuse accusations directed at parents of children with OI come about because neither parents nor accusers know of the condition's existence. In cases where the diagnosis of OI occurs at birth, the parents know their child has the condition and act accordingly. This lessens the risk that they will be falsely accused of abuse. In many cases, however, children with OI are not yet diagnosed, and since fractures can happen spontaneously, neither the parents nor the child can satisfactorily explain why the fracture occurred. This can generate suspicions among teachers, doctors, and others who have a duty to report possible cases of abuse. Combine these factors with the "guilty until proven innocent" attitude among many who investigate child-abuse cases, and many parents find themselves in a legalistic and bureaucratic nightmare.

Diagnosis

Usually false accusations of child abuse occur in families with children who have milder forms of OI and in whom OI had not previously been diagnosed. The scenario is ripe for misdiagnosis.

- The parents have an unlikely, or unsatisfactory, or no explanation of how the fracture occurred.
- X-rays reveal other, possibly unreported fractures in various stages of healing
- Bruising is sometimes evident
- The bones appear otherwise normal on X-rays
- The child appears normal

It has been said that by looking at X-rays, OI can be distinguished from child abuse. Unfortunately, we have learned that the differential diagnosis is not that rudimentary. Types of fractures that are typically observed in both child abuse and OI include:

- fractures in multiple stages of healing
- rib fractures
- spiral fractures
- fractures for which there is no adequate explanation of trauma

When the fracture seems incompatible with the severity of injury, child abuse is generally considered. For example, most children do not break a bone by falling out of bed. Yet, making that determination based upon the credibility of the caregiver's report of how the accident occurred can lead to erroneous conclusions. Unfortunately, in most OI fractures, the cause of the fracture is almost always inconsistent with the trauma.

Joffe and Ludwig,[2] reported that of 363 children that fell down stairways, only 6% of these children had fractures. And in the same report, of 85 hospital incident reports involving falls of children under five years of age there was only one fracture. However, if a single child with OI were to fall down a stairway, the likelihood of the fall resulting in numerous severe fractures is great.

Medical professionals have been known to rule out OI when clinical manifestations such as blue sclerae or opalescent teeth, symptomatic X-rays, or family histories of OI are lacking, and the physical appearance of the child is normal. Yet, often, children with the milder forms of OI do not demonstrate these commonly recognized symptoms and features. Those who are often mistaken as having been victims of child abuse are the most difficult to diagnose as having OI.

Collagen testing, a relatively new means of diagnosing OI leaves at least a 10-15% margin of error. This means that while collagen testing will identify the majority of people who have OI, approximately 10-15% of individuals who actually do have OI will test negative, and therefore, are not detected through collagen testing. Also, for families already traumatized by false accusations of child abuse, and possibly enduring the distress of their child being removed from the home by Child Protection Services, the 6 - 8 week waiting period for test results can seem like an eternity.

One experienced OI Foundation Child Abuse Counselor recommends that parents who have been wrongfully accused of child abuse opt not to undergo collagen testing. Because an inconclusive finding is considered negative by many Child Protection Service Departments, a questionable diagnosis is often more damaging than no diagnosis at all. In some cases, a clinical diagnosis from a physician who is very knowledgeable about OI leads to a more reliable conclusion.

Volunteers at the Osteogenesis Imperfecta Foundation are working diligently to increase public and professional awareness about this problem. In 1990, a project funded by Ronald McDonald Children's Charities disseminated educational material to nearly 60,000 health care professionals, social welfare agencies, hospitals, libraries, and media health editors in an effort to increase awareness about the problem of parents of children with OI being erroneously accused of child abuse. Yet still, every year parents of children with OI are wrongly accused of abusing their children. It is important to remember that society has an interest in protecting its children, and often this interest clashes with the rights of parents. Until a balance is struck between the two, the best way to reduce the number of false accusations within the OI community is to make the existence of OI common knowledge within the larger community.

Unfortunately, when false accusations of child abuse occur, families become victimized. The following advice is intended to help parents resolve such situations by cooperating as fully as they can with the authorities investigating them.

Guidelines for families of children with OI who are wrongfully suspected of child abuse

- Remember that case workers are only doing their jobs and that whoever reported this is bound by law to do so. No one is really "out to get you."
- Seek the best medical diagnosis available. It is of utmost importance that the person conducting the evaluation have considerable experience in both treating and diagnosing OI. Often, local orthopaedic surgeons are only experienced in treating very severe cases of OI, and will not validate a mild case as truly being OI.
- A consultation with a geneticist familiar with OI may reveal a family history of mild OI if symptoms such as presenile hearing loss, rickets, dental problems and short stature are identified.
- Keep the case worker up to date on what is happening. Prove you are not enemies with this person, but indeed want to work together for what is best for your child. Resistance toward the case worker may be interpreted as guilt.
- You may request that the child not be taken from the home. State your willingness to work with a "support program" for abusive parents while still seeking a diagnosis for the child. It is very important to be cooperative even though you are not guilty. If the child is being taken from the home, you may request that he or she be taken to the home of a grandparent or other relative.
- Each state has its own policy on dealing with child abuse cases. We suggest you secure the services of an attorney if the matter is not resolved quickly.
- Most often, child abuse is suspected when the explanation given by the child or parent does not match the injury found by the medical staff, and decisions are based heavily on the medical information given the agency by the doctor.
- When the problem is resolved, insist that the charges be taken off all records including computerized records. If this is not done, you will be registered as an abusive parent until your youngest child is 18 years of age.

Endnotes

1. **Feibusch, Kate**, *Handle with Care: Is it really child abuse? The Pharos of Alpha Omega Alpha Honor Medical Society*, Winter 1993:34-36.
2. **Joffe, M., Ludwig, S.**, *Stairway injuries in children. Pediatrics*, 1988; 82:457-461.

DECIDE FOR YOURSELF...
IS THIS AN ABUSED CHILD?

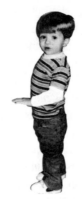

A traumatized child

Unlikely or unsatisfactory
explanation of how the
fracture occurred

X-rays that reveal old
fractures in various stages
of healing

Evidence of Bruising

Varied types of fractures

Bones that appear
normal on X-rays

NO, This child, like hundreds of children thought to have been abused, actually
has Osteogenesis Imperfecta or Brittle Bone Disorder. At his current age of 10
he has experienced over 65 fractures. In distinguishing between child abuse and
OI there are similarities, but please be aware of the important differences.*

- Blue Sclera, (whites of the eyes)
- Inverted triangular shaped skull
- Small stature
- Excessive mobility of the joints
- Thin fragile skin

- Excessive sweating
- Little soft tissue damage at fracture site
- Crush fractures of the vertebrae
- X-rays that reveal wormian bones
- Discolored, breakable teeth

*It is important to note that few patients with Osteogenesis Imperfecta (OI) show
all of the listed abnormalities, and some show *none*. Some children with OI outwardly appear normal in every respect. A diagnostic test for OI in the form of a
skin biopsy is available. It requires approximately 3 months to obtain results.

For more information, contact:

Chapter 18

Unique Concerns of People with Milder OI

By Carole Hagin
Martinez, California

I look like an average 59 year old woman. I am married, am an active mother of seven grown children, and grandmother to eight. I work twelve hour shifts at a local hospital, and though I was unaware of it until recently, I have mild osteogenesis imperfecta.

I discovered my OI at age 52 at the University of California Medical Center where an endocrinologist whom I'll call "Sherlock Holmes", actually listened to the many mysterious complaints that had been plaguing my body for most of my life. As I aged, my vague and unexplainable complaints seemed to worsen and then escalate at menopause. In 1986, I was referred to the University of California, San Francisco by my oral surgeon, who expressed concern about the quality of the bones in my jaw during surgery. A lifetime of concerns were addressed by the endocrinologist who deciphered the clues I gave, ordered the right lab tests, and solved my case with a diagnosis of mild osteogenesis imperfecta. As I learn more about OI, my concerns and symptoms now have an explanation, and I am very relieved to find a place for them.

Through my own experiences, and through conversations I have enjoyed with other people with type I, or milder OI, consistent concerns arise and certain problems seem to be unique to our milder form of OI. I would like to address some of these concerns in the pages that follow.

Delayed Diagnosis

Obtaining timely and accurate diagnoses of and information about mild OI is often very difficult. Physicians are often unfamiliar with the vague and confusing symptoms presented to them. When people with mild OI do not have a name or an explanation for the many complaints and problems they experience, a low self image can develop. Young

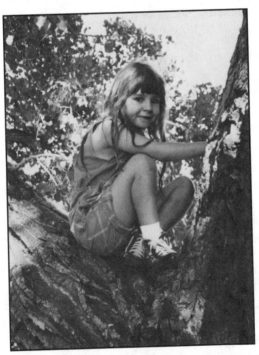

people who do not know they have OI often feel small and fragile. A different physical appearance, with no explanation of why, can lead to feelings of peculiarity and separation from peers. They may wonder why they hurt a lot, and fear being seen as complainers. Often, aches and pains are kept confidential to avoid the reputation of being a whiner.

Sometimes people with mild OI experience years of unexplained fractures before a diagnosis of OI is even considered. Often, injuries are sustained due to participation in activities that might have been deemed inappropriate, had it been known that OI existed. It was most disconcerting to one of my high school dates to find that an exuberant hug broke three of my ribs. Not knowing about OI, I was puzzled by the ease with which I could fracture. I hated the way this could limit my way of life.

False Accusations of Child Abuse

Parents of children with the milder forms of OI are generally those who are wrongfully accused of child abuse. Many physicians, when they hear the words osteogenesis imperfecta, think first of the more severe forms of OI. For some, it seems incomprehensible that a child, who appears average in many respects, could possibly have the severely debilitating disorder mentioned briefly in the medical textbooks. Because of this, parents of children with the milder forms of OI become the victims of false accusations of child abuse and endure unfortunate mistreatment and misfortune at the hands of well-meaning social workers and medical professionals.

It is extremely important for parents of children with the milder forms of OI to obtain a letter of identification to confirm diagnosis of OI should a question arise. Especially when traveling, this precaution becomes even more critical.

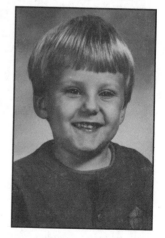

Looking "Normal" and Feeling Brittle

Another difficulty, especially unique to children with the milder forms of OI, is that of desperately wanting to "be like the other kids", but being physically unable to "keep up with the pack". Many children with milder OI appear like their peers in most respects. But with physical abilities that may be delayed, keeping up with neighborhood or school friends can become a frustrating and disheartening obstacle.

Lack of Awareness About OI within the Medical Profession

The lack of professional knowledge about OI is even more evident when it comes to milder OI. Among those medical professionals who are aware of OI, many are only familiar with the more severe forms.

When OI exists but is yet undiagnosed, a visit to the doctor's office can be very invalidating. Years of frustration, unanswered questions, and a lack of appropriate treatment become disheartening. A fracture that does not show up on an initial x-ray can be diagnosed as a sprain or strain, and be treated inappropriately.

Aches

Many people with milder OI experience years of unexplained

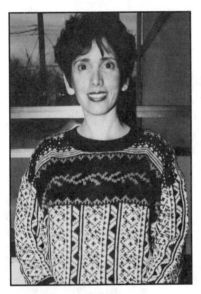

aches and pains. Pain in the long bones and ribs are sometimes described as 'growing pains''. Often pain is initially caused by undiagnosed fractures. Later in life, arthritis, scoliosis, and stiffness can make beneficial exercise difficult or can lead to even more pain.

Dental Concerns and Hearing Loss

The dental and oral concerns of people with mild OI seem to be similar to those experienced by people with the other forms of OI. A person with OI type 1A will have unaffected teeth, whereas a person with OI type 1B will have affected teeth or opalescent dentin.

People with the milder forms of OI are more likely to experience pre-senile hearing loss. Treatment for hearing loss associated with OI can usually be effectively treated as described elsewhere in this book.

Heredity and Genetic Counseling

Type IA or 1B OI is autosomal dominant, allowing for a fifty percent chance of having a child also affected by OI. Often, people with milder OI do not seek genetic counseling prior to the start of their

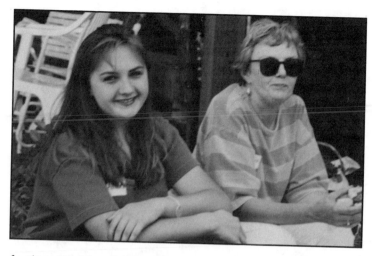

families. I have heard the thought expressed, "OI was never a big inconvenience in my life. If my offspring experience consequences as insignificant as mine, then why bother with genetic counseling?" Although it is generally true that a child will inherit the same level of severity of OI as their affected parent, it is also possible for the child to experience a more severe case. Genetic counseling can be valuable to any family with a history of any type of OI.

Conclusion

I value this body, even if it is achy and at times disabled, I will continue to care for it. I know I am fortunate to be able to ambulate and work easily, even when OI becomes visible. People with the milder forms of OI are encouraged to provide support to each other through local contacts, support groups, and through the Osteogenesis Imperfecta Foundation national conferences. Together, we can equate our experiences of being "just a little brittle."

Works Cited

Notelovitz, Morris, M.D., and Ware, Marsha, *Stand Tall! Every Woman's Guide to Preventing Osteoporosis, Bantam Books, 1984.*

Fardon, David M., M.D., *Osteoporosis, Your Head Start on the Prevention and Treatment of Brittle Bones. The Body Press, 1987.*

Marini, Joan, M.D., Ph.D., *Osteogenesis Imperfecta: Clinical Types and Genetics, Feb, 1986.*

Paterson, Colin R., McAllion, Susan, Stellman, Joan L., *Osteogenesis Imperfecta After the Menopause, New England Journal of Medicine. 1984, 3310:1694-6.*

Chapter 19

Independent Living

by Kathy Collins
Helena, Montana

A child is ready and expected to leave home upon becoming an adult. Most parents take this fact of life for granted. This cherished rite of passage, however, is often deemed impossible by the parents of children with OI. Often parents refuse to believe there is any way their child could function independently outside the home. Moreover, the misgivings of parents are often surpassed by the fears held by the person with OI himself. Yet, in recent years, more and more people with even severe OI have begun living independently, their fears having become increasingly unwarranted.

The Independent Living Movement

In the 1960s, a group of students with severe disabilities at the University of California at Berkeley identified their own similar needs for independence: accessible transportation; reliable personal care attendants to assist with daily needs such as bathing, getting in and out of bed, dressing and cooking; and affordable, accessible housing. Together they devised a system that provided for these needs and, through grant writing and intensive lobbying and much effort, the first Center for Independent Living was born.

Independence for persons with disabilities was furthered by Congress through the 1973 passage of the Rehabilitation Act. Part B of this act set aside funds specifically earmarked for the establishment of regional independent living centers. Each center's approach to independent living was as unique as the people it served. Some offered personal care attendants, accessible transportation systems, LPN services, housing or referrals to accessible housing, employment training, and recreational opportunities. Others developed comprehensive peer counseling services and independent living skills training.

As deinstitutionalization of people with disabilities became more prevalent, the centers began to offer additional services to persons with wider ranges of disabilities. From the largest cities to the most sparsely populated rural areas, these consumer controlled centers helped ease the way for people with disabilities to live independently.

By law, the majority of board members of the independent living centers must be persons with disabilities. Although board members are not involved in the day-to-day business of the center, they set policies and procedures and plan for future programs. Members play a variety of roles, from advocates to consultants to consumers of the center's services.

Finances

One of the toughest aspects of moving out on one's own, disabled or not, has to do with money; or, more importantly, how to acquire sufficient funds to live comfortably. Programs and information about financial security are available through local Social Security offices. If a person with OI qualifies for SSI, (Supplemental Security Income), or SSDI, (Social Security Disability Insurance), he or she may also qualify for Medicaid and/or Medicare. However, people who have tried to live on these programs know too well the frustration of "spend downs" and the myriad of rules and regulations that a $425-a-month SSI check can bring. Often people with OI who are dependent on government aid become locked into lives with very low incomes.

How is the chain of poverty broken? Through education, of course. Just as members of the non-disabled community can remove themselves and their families from the low-income rut, so can those with OI. High schools are becoming keenly aware that not all students are college bound. Vocational training in a variety of fields is standard in most school districts. For those who choose to seek a college education, Vocational Rehabilitation programs can provide counseling, training, and funding for education. More colleges and universities have become sensitive to the needs of the disabled student providing accessible housing, interpreters for the hearing impaired, and making appropriate accommodations for those with mobility impairments.

Since most people with OI are of average or above-average intelligence, seeking higher education in fields that correlate with their unique talents will ultimately provide the highest probability for financial security. By preparing for professional positions and taking advantage of programs available in Vocational Rehabilitation, people with OI open the doors to opportunity and prepare themselves financially for independent living.

Housing

In theory, today's housing market is much different than it was 20 years ago. Many builders are now concerned with accessibility standards in new and existing housing. The Americans with Disabilities Act has also provided people with the legal protection they need to secure suitable housing. In practice, however, the situation is usually much different.

Rental housing is often inaccessible to wheelchairs. Doorways may be too narrow,

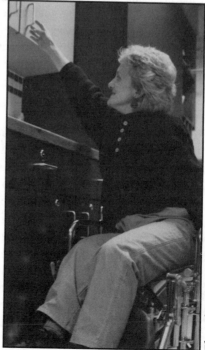

Photo by Laura Vincheal

countertops too high, bathrooms too small, and landlords unwilling to modify their property to meet the needs of a tenant with OI. When searching for an apartment, check local want ads, set up appointments, and have an able-bodied assistant willing to help you look. Don't be discouraged if you encounter sites where accessibility has been assured, but you learn otherwise. True accessibility is a hard concept for many people to grasp.

Buying a house poses entirely different problems. Remodeling for accessibility can add substantially to the cost of a home. The payoff, of course, lies in having a home made to meet your exact needs. If you do not have sufficient funds to make all of the accommodations at once, prioritize your needs and then remodel as money permits. If you are able to build a new home, be sure to choose a builder who truly knows accessible architecture and who is willing to listen and accommodate special needs that are requested. With the builder, brainstorm your "wish list" of options for the new home. Also, talk to others who have built to their specifications and find out what they would have done differently, keeping in mind that everyone's needs are unique.

Not all people with OI need to leave the family home in order to live independently. Some families are willing and financially able to set up private accommodations and convenience apartments within the home or on their property. Living a bit removed from the family circle allows more freedom and control and provides greater opportunity for independence. Sometimes it helps to move toward independence gradually, and these measures can help.

Personal Care Needs

Some people with severe OI require help with bathing, dressing, getting in and out of bed, cooking, cleaning, and other personal tasks. Most communities across the country have identified these services as necessary not only for the disabled but also for the elderly. Nevertheless, most people can be cared for comfortably and safely in their own homes through the use of home health service providers. The U.S. government and insurance companies learned years ago that it is much more cost-effective to pay for personal care attendant (PCA) services in the home than to house the disabled and elderly in nursing homes. For people with OI who have more acute care needs, such as respirator dependence, LPN and RN care is also an option.

It's not uncommon for a person with OI who has been accustomed to being provided with significant assistance in daily living to have no idea of how to manage on his or her own. Because of this, many independent living centers provide independent living skills training. Usually this process begins with an assessment of the person's skill level, followed by an individualized training program. These programs may teach the person how to cook, manage a budget, shop for groceries, and do housekeeping. Training sessions are set up to meet the disabled person's individual needs, taking their particular situations into account.

Housekeeping tasks such as vacuuming and mopping floors can be done by professional housekeepers. Meal preparation can be made easier by purchasing frozen dinners or ready-made foods in the deli section of the supermarket. For the truly energetic, large meals can be prepared and then sectioned off into individual servings to be frozen and used later. Whatever the choice, it's important to be sure to consider all the options.

Some people with OI have chosen to obtain a "service dog" to assist with independent living skills. Similar to "seeing eye dogs" for the blind, service dogs are trained to provide assistance for people with disabilities. Tasks such as pulling wheelchairs, turning off and on light switches, opening heavy doors, and reaching hard-to-reach items are accomplished by these loving companions.

Transportation

Transportation opportunities are increasing for persons with OI. Specialized transit systems in the past were costly and used most often to transport patients from nursing homes to doctor's offices or hospitals. Now, local

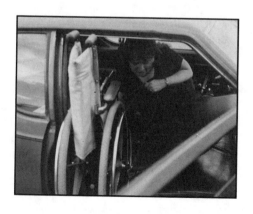

transit systems are required by law to accommodate the disabled. Some systems provide access on modified buses that can accommodate wheelchairs and persons with mobility impairments. Although some communities are allowed as much as ten years to comply with these regulations, for the most part some sort of accessibility is available nationwide. Taxi companies are beginning to cash in on this market by purchasing vehicles with lifts or ramps. Car manufacturers are offering rebates to those who purchase a vehicle that needs to be specially modified. Transportation trends are definitely taking the needs of people with disabilities into consideration.

Mini-vans have become the answer to a wheelchair user's prayers. Not only are they much more fuel efficient than their larger counter-

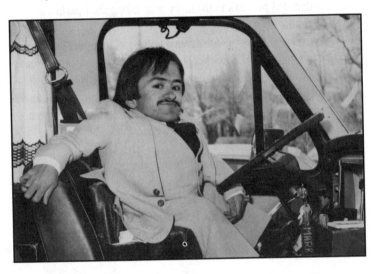

parts, they offer a variety of modification options. Some features are complex and costly while others are quite simple. Whether the vehicle is to be driven by the person with OI or by an attendant, the options are increasing all the time.

Selections in automobile hand controls have grown lately, too. Some models allow for both accelerator and brakes to be operated with a single control next to the steering wheel. Other sets may be adapted for a person who is short statured who may simply need the pedals extended. Medical supply companies generally offer information on a variety of manufacturers of hand controls. Seating modifications can be adjusted then as well.

Employment

Job hunting can be an extremely difficult task for anyone. Nothing can wrinkle the self-esteem like trying to look for work. Resumes and presenting oneself in the best light possible are extremely important sales tools for someone looking for employment. Many local job service offices offer classes to individuals looking for work and can provide helpful pointers to people new to the job market. Vocational Rehabilitation offices also offer formal job seeking information for disabled people who qualify.

In seeking employment, it's important for people with OI to know their rights and to seek positions for which they are qualified. Tax incentives are available to employers who hire disabled workers and these incentives can help pay for any expenses incurred to make the employment site more accessible. Be sure to learn the laws established to protect the rights of the disabled.

Unfortunately, prejudice still exists in this country regarding hiring people with disabilities. Many employers do not perceive disabled applicants as capable of doing a job; therefore, it becomes the task of the disabled person to educate and reassure the prospective employer. As more people with disabilities become employed and visible in the job market, the road becomes easier for those who follow. But now, people with disabilities must do exceptional jobs of selling themselves and their skills.

Peer Counseling

Talking with someone with experience in any endeavor you plan to pursue is always very valuable. For a person with OI interested in learning to live independently, a peer counseling program can be a great help. Available at most Independent Living Centers, a peer counseling program matches a trained peer with a disability with a person who is recently disabled or just beginning to live independently. Peer helpers must undergo hours of training to give them skills necessary in assisting someone else with a disability. These programs may vary a little from one center to the next, but most of them give support systems to those who may need it at critical times in their lives.

Emergencies, or what if the worst happens?

It never hurts to prepare for the worst because sometimes, as people with OI have learned, the worst can happen. It's extremely important for someone with O.I. to have an emergency plan worked out before emergencies happen. Not only can fractures occur, but wheelchair batteries can go dead, vans can break down and lifts can malfunction, among other calamities.

Phones should have automatic dialing for police, fire, and ambulance, along with the numbers of people in your life who live close by and can help if you get in a jam. In the case of a fracture, especially, it is important to have friends or relatives who know what to do and can accompany you to the emergency room if necessary. An emergency device with a direct connection to 911 can be set up through the phone.

Planning for the future

It is important for parents of children with OI to insist that their child participate in family chores. Sometimes the state of fractures and the severity of OI may prevent some tasks from being done. However, it is extremely important for the children to be prepared for some level of independence. Meal planning, dish-washing, folding laundry, grocery shopping, pet care, making lunch sandwiches, etc., are basic chores. Insisting that a child with OI participate in these activities not only prepares them for adult independence, but it builds self-esteem in knowing he or she can be an active, contributing member of the family.

Living isn't just something that happens to us; it's something we make happen ourselves. For a child with OI, learning how to live independently begins long before the child ever steps out on his or her own. For the child's parents, teaching those skills - and learning how to let go - begins just as early.

Chapter 20

Deciding to Become a Parent

By Heidi C. Glauser, Pittsburgh, Pennsylvania and Deborah Yarborough, Santa Clara, California

"Having OI, or any disability, should never stop a person from fulfilling their life goals and desires. And especially OI should not keep a person from something as important and fulfilling as having a family. OI is not that big of a deal. We break, we get better. So what?" (Laurie Driscoll)

How will OI affect my ability to be a parent?

A person's attitude about having OI plays an important role in determining how OI will affect that person's ability to be a parent. As in other areas of life, someone with a positive and optimistic personal attitude about having OI will find parenting to be a fulfilling, challenging, and most rewarding experience. On the other hand, a person with a negative attitude about having OI, or one who might convey a message such as, "Poor me," or "The world owes me," or "How can you expect me to function, can't you see I have OI," might consider parenthood to be an overwhelming, burdensome task.

For this essay, ten adults with OI were interviewed. According to all ten, first thoughts about parenthood occurred during the late teen years or early twenties. Prior to that time, only those with mild OI received encouragement to consider parenthood from family or friends. Those with more severe forms of OI reported it rare to hear statements, commonly expressed to able-bodied children, such as "When you become a mommy...," or "I know you'll be a great dad some day." Within one family, a young woman with OI ignored the counsel she received as a child, that said since she would never get married, she "had better learn to type." This woman has since married and is currently the proud and successful mother of four charming children. Serious consideration of parenthood by people with the more severe forms of OI generally surfaced first between husband and wife during the early years of marriage.

Should we adopt or have biological children?

When one or both spouses have OI, the question of adoption or having biological children frequently arises. Some couples sought the advice of a genetic counselor to learn about the likelihood of future

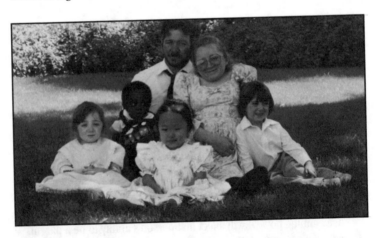

children inheriting OI. For others knowing the chances of having a child with OI was not a factor. Their goal was simply to begin a family. Whether their child was born with or without OI was irrelevant.

Although most couples discussed their options with family members and friends, the most helpful advice came from other parents with OI or parents with other disabilities, especially various forms of short stature. Many adults with OI have benefitted from discussions generated at the Osteogenesis Imperfecta Foundation or Little People of America national conferences. Within these valuable forums, adults can freely discuss parenting options with others who have evaluated the alternatives and decided upon a course of action.

Adoption

Many factors enter into a couple's decision to adopt or give birth to a biological child. What follows is a list of considerations expressed by people with OI who choose adoption over having biological children:

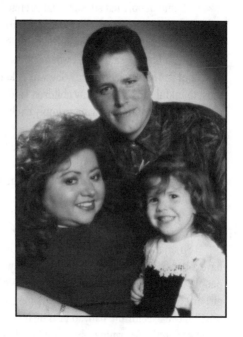

- We chose adoption because we prefer not to pass OI along to our children.
- Caring for a child with OI would be too difficult considering the physical limitations of OI.
- The adoption of an able-bodied child who would facilitate his or her own ability to be independently mobile is an advantage.
- Knowing that there are children with OI or other disabilities already born and in need of loving homes, we choose to adopt these special children.
- For some women with OI, the actual requirements of bearing a child exceed the body's physiological ability.
- The extent of the physical toll upon the body of the woman with OI is often unpredictable and thus unacceptable.

Having Biological Children

Some adults with OI, when contemplating the choices for parenthood, have considered artificial insemination or egg donation. As Andrew Yarborough stated, "I never considered the contribution of genetic material to be a prerequisite for fatherhood." And his wife Debbie states, "We also considered inviting a family member to act as a surrogate parent, but concluded that the emotional complications associated with that avenue were prohibitive." None of those surveyed opted to pursue these alternative paths.

Some people felt strongly that prenatal screening for OI be used only as a means to identify the most appropriate method for birth, ie. vaginal or caesarian section. Nine-year-old Rianna Driscoll, whose mother also has OI, said it best when she participated in a questionnaire in school at Thanksgiving time. She was asked to report what she was most thankful for. While many children said they were thankful for their parents, or their homes, Rianna simply exclaimed, "Above all, I am thankful for my life."

In contrast, some adults with OI believe that they, as potential parents, should seek prenatal counseling for the purpose of factoring that information into their decision about their own willingness and capabilities to be parents of a child with OI.

Does is matter if my child has OI?

So often, it's heard when a new baby is born, "We don't care if we have a boy or a girl, we just hope it's healthy." In contrast, for some people with OI, the expression could be, "We don't care if it's a boy or a girl or even if it's 'healthy.'" When the parent has OI, and a strong possibility exists for the baby to also be born with OI, the parents together should determine whether a "healthy" child is hoped for, or if the issue is even relevant to them.

When the occurrence of OI is not an issue, parents bypass the disappointment experienced by many able-bodied parents when they learn that their infant has OI. Laurie Driscoll states, "Having a child with OI was not a fear, nor did we secretly hope to have a "healthy" baby. I knew since age 13 that some day I would have a little girl, and she would be just like me. When my little girl was born, all was right. I never thought that having OI was something bad or to be avoided. Different, yes, but very right for me."

Laurie continues, "In truth, my son without OI is more challenging to me in many ways. At the time of his birth, his grandmother exclaimed, 'We're so glad he's normal.' But to me, an able-bodied child is abnormal. Children with OI are normal. How to cope with this able-bodied very physical son is, in many ways more demanding and 'unnatural' than parenting my children with OI."

Barbie Simmonds, who has Type I OI, states, "While growing up, broken bones were normal in our family. The idea of having a child with OI never scared me, I guess because I never viewed it as a liability."

Medical feasibility - Can my body carry a child?

Many women with OI must be concerned about the physical toll that pregnancy and motherhood can exert upon her body. Debbie Yarborough, who is currently considering parenthood, states, "No one knows my body better than I do, and as I imagined the changes my body would go through in bearing a child to term, even with caesarian section birth, I would likely do injury to myself, and possibly impair my ability to walk ... and care for my child and our home. The tradeoffs were not worth the risks."

Is parenthood and OI compatible?

One of the primary concerns of parents with OI is the physical limitations that prohibit full interaction with their child. Pat Lang, whose husband, Ed, also has OI, states, "When our children were babies we did a lot of adapting to our height, physical abilities, and strength. Once they were walking and able to climb in and out of car seats and high chairs, it was much easier. Children raised at an early age with OI parents seem to sense ... their parent's limitations."

Sally Franklin, who is three feet tall and the parent of a biological daughter without OI, states, "I learned a lot of tricks to rearing an infant. I had to compensate for not being able to 'lug' my child and I had to secure her as a toddler so she did not venture into dangerous situations."

One's anticipated longevity is rarely considered when contemplating the life-long commitment of parenthood. Pat Lang reports, "My husband Ed had a stroke recently and is now in a nursing home needing total physical care. I now, at age 48, have total responsibility for the children, home, and Ed's care. Now more than ever I thank God for the children. They are my life. My only fear is keeping my own health."

When necessary, many parents with OI develop and come to rely upon a close network of loved ones and friends. Barbie Simmonds states, "I would not do anything differently [concerning my choice to have a child with OI], but I am facing many parenting issues that I never realized would surface."

Being a parent with OI has many positive features:

- "I value my child's achievements on their own merit, not based on comparisons with others." (Simmonds)
- "I am proud that Kimberly will grow up ... fully aware of just how 'able' people with disabilities are. She will see that we have little room for excuses in what we can accomplish." (Williams)
- "It's great to be little in a room full of children. I find they relate to me so easily because I am their size, at their level, and they gravitate towards that." (Driscoll)

Dealing with Fractures and Pain

"I wouldn't be honest if I said that I never question our decision to give birth to children with OI. When I witness the pain that my children experience when a fracture occurs, or after a surgery, it's real difficult. When Rianna started breaking, I experienced real "guilt"; maybe not guilt, but it was hard to accept emotionally. A strong religious view of the importance of life helps me a lot."

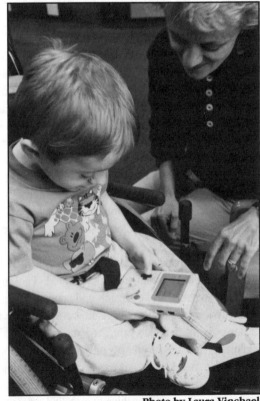

Laurie, who has one biological daughter with OI, a biological son without OI,

Photo by Laura Vinchael

and two adopted children with OI, continues, "When one of my adopted children break something, I find it to be less difficult than when my biological child fractures. Perhaps it is because the adopted children were older when they came to live with us, and that initial bond developed later, or perhaps it is because with Rianna I know her OI came from me. With the two adopted children, I can cast, straighten, and take care of their fractures. But when Rianna breaks, I cannot do the hard stuff. It seems harder because of the different relationship I have between my birth and adopted children."

Summary

Children born to parents with OI can grow to be positive, social, and happy children when parents instill that optimism in them from a young age. Both the avenues of adoption and having biological children are being successfully assumed by adults with OI. Some parents opt not to bring a child into the world with OI – while others believe that having a child with OI is not to be avoided. Consideration of the medical feasibility of carrying a child is of critical importance to women with OI considering motherhood. Although physical limitations are frustrating for many parents with OI, most are convinced that their children are not missing anything critical because of their OI. On the contrary, many positive characteristics, attributable to OI attest to the fact that parenthood and OI are generally compatible.

> *"Having OI is no reason to be depressed. When a bone breaks the hard part is not that you broke, but what part of life you'll miss because of the fracture. So certainly we should not consciously put restrictions upon ourselves and let ourselves miss out on any aspect of life when we don't have to."* (Driscoll)

Special thanks to the following people who contributed their personal perspectives to this essay through questionnaires and interviews.

Scott and Laurie Driscoll, Mesa, Arizona
Sally Franklin, Bozeman, Montana
Ed and Pat Lang, Miami, Florida
Barbie Simmonds, Arlington, Virginia
Bill and Marsha Williams, Nicholasville, Kentucky
Andrew and Debbie Yarborough, Santa Clara, California

Chapter 21

Severe Osteogenesis Imperfecta - The First Weeks of Life

by Grace A. Sisco
Easter Seal Society of Utah
Salt Lake City, Utah

Many children with severe OI enter the world perilously. The first weeks of life become critical for both the child and the parents. Children born with type II and severe type III OI often need adept handling, decisive treatment, and particular care. I speak to parents and others who require insight on how to care for these fragile yet valiant newborns.

As medicine becomes more successful in prolonging the lives of children born with very severe OI, unique concerns surface. Parents soon learn to draw upon information and support derived from other parents. Although other parents will not have all the answers, there is comfort in knowing that you are not alone.

A Model of Perspective

To gain an understanding of the future for you and your child is at best, difficult. The following model, (Fig. 21-1), displays four factors that can influence the future of the infant with severe OI. The four intersecting circles represent:

- the severity of the child's OI
- "wellness" - health potentials such as survival instincts, immunities, etc.
- the environment

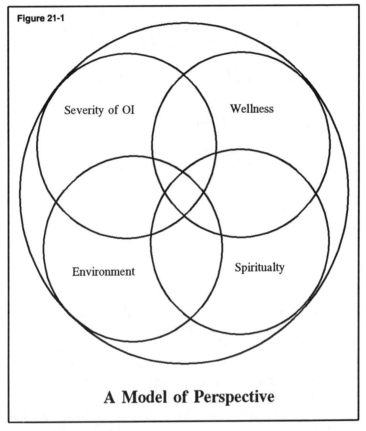

Figure 21-1

A Model of Perspective

- spirituality or religion

The complexity of these factors, separate and in combination, may influence the baby's chance of survival. Over some aspects, you have no control, such as the severity of the OI. You can exert a degree of influence over other aspects, such as wellness, and finally, there are aspects within the baby's environment, over which you can exert control and have significant impact on your baby's future.

Getting the News

Initially, you may be given a flurry of medical and genetic information. Depending upon the resources and expertise of the birth hospital, this information may be complete or severely lacking. A lack of accurate information can be very bewildering and difficult for parents. It is important to remember that neither parent did anything to cause OI to occur. Speculation about the source of your baby's OI, as being due to the environment, circumstances during pregnancy, or possibly a relative, is natural but generally irrelevant. When no family history of OI exists, its occurrence can rarely be attributed to a cause over which you may have had control.

Many times the physician will present the worst case scenario, or predict a slim chance of survival for your baby. The information provided may be offensive or hurtful to you. When faced with a difficult diagnosis, physicians are sometimes unsure of how to best approach a family. Some parents, in their frustration and devastation have lashed out at the "messenger". It is important to acknowledge your own emotional stress, and to retain an objective attitude toward health care providers and the information they provide. There is much you must learn from them.

To learn that some infants born with severe OI eventually do thrive and lead fulfilling lives, can fuel the hope necessary for the demanding weeks ahead. Information, referrals, and assistive devices to optimize your baby's chances of survival and enhanced quality of life become most appreciated. Most often the needed balance of

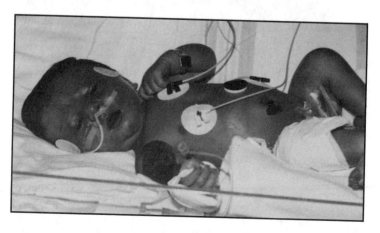

information can be obtained through the Osteogenesis Imperfecta Foundation in written material, videos, and most importantly, through the parent support network. It is important to reach out for this balance of information as soon as possible.

The uncertainty of not knowing what the future will hold can be very frustrating to new parents who want desperately to know what will happen to their child. But because of the great variation in the symptoms and manifestations of OI, it is important not to generalize or make assumptions about how your child will fare based upon what is seen in others you may contact.

Information is Power

Knowledge is your best tool and can also be very therapeutic. Gather and read as much information and data as possible. At first, you will probably be looking for answers to immediate and specific concerns. It may be months or even years before you actually digest all the information about OI that is initially available.

Parents often utilize different coping mechanisms. Remember

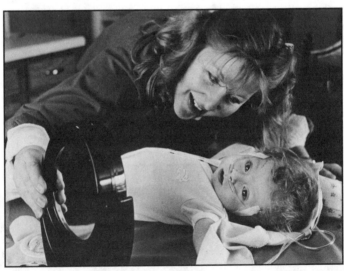

Photo by Gerald Silver

that you will not necessarily see the problems and prognosis the same as your spouse. Effective communication between parents is essential in the care of your child.

Developing a Bond with Your Child

Initially, you may hesitate to bond with a child that may not survive. Well-meaning relatives or friends may caution you against being too hopeful. You may not even realize that you are withholding natural emotions, especially if the baby is your first. This initial bonding plays an important part in your baby's wellness and should be developed.

Believe in life no matter what. Focus on closeness, stimulation, and giving your child the love he or she needs to survive. Methods such as singing to the child, gently stroking, and helping the child to recognize the parents unique smell by putting Mom or Dads pillowcase into the crib can all aid in developing this important bond.

Even children with very severe OI do survive if all factors work in their favor. Don't be afraid to love and hope freely. Even families who have lost a child with a severe disability cherish memories, embrace the love they have felt, and appreciate the personal growth experienced. Even after losing a loved baby, parents recover and go on with life, whole and healthy. Yes, with sadness and feelings of great loss, but knowing they loved and did their best to give their child a chance.

Becoming Your Child's Case Manager

Many hospitals and/or state Health Departments have case managers assigned to babies with disabilities and their families. A case manager is the person who will oversee and coordinate the care and decision making for the child and his/her family. Provided as part of federal early intervention programs, case managers are sometimes offered upon discharge from the hospital. Due to the rarity and lack of general knowledge about OI, often a parent chooses to becomes his child's own case manager.

Services specifically for the child are called early intervention programs. Respite services are for the family as a whole. State offices of health and/or human services, nonprofit agencies such as Easter Seal Societies, or private firms such as rehabilitation hospitals and medical supply companies may all offer services in your area.

Major Medical Decision-making

Sometimes you will be required to make important decisions regarding the amount and type of medical intervention utilized in behalf of your child. After hearing the counsel of the medical staff, parents should come to an agreement about their wishes, and then communicate these desires in writing to the medical staff. To not be prepared for these situations is to turn control over to the medical staff

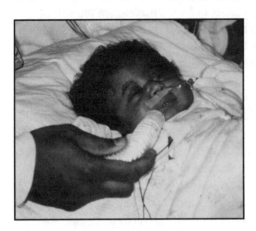

who may choose a treatment that is more or less aggressive than the choice you would have made. It is also acceptable to not make these decisions if you cannot. If an order, such as a "do not resuscitate", is made in writing, make sure these instructions are reviewed and rewritten or discarded as your child's health and prognosis changes.

Complications experienced by newborns with OI can include respiratory failure, hemorrhaging, hernias and, of course, fractures. Sometimes surgical procedures can improve difficulties encountered. It may help for you to obtain from other parents the names of physicians experienced in treating children with OI.

Treatment of Fractures

When multiple fractures occur during birth, splinting can ease the pain and allow the baby to focus on the need for rest and nutrition. Often bone structure is so poor that fractures are not visible on x-rays. Some parents choose not to take the child to the doctor or emergency room for every break, but learn to apply a splint at home. Together with your child, it becomes possible to determine when to seek medical attention for a fracture and when it is best to wait. Some children with severe OI may actually experience fewer major fractures but complain of continuous micro fractures. If deformities exist that impair the ability of your child to sit, surgical correction should be considered as soon as possible.

Handling the Severely Affected Infant

At times it is best to limit the handling of a baby with multiple fractures. Some babies may not tolerate laying on flat surfaces or even on a flat crib mattress. An alternative is to use a pillow or egg crate foam inside a pillow case. Another suggestion is to utilize an infant bathtub supplied with handles. The sides on the bathtub prevent the baby from rolling, and the foam insert can be cut and customized to fit. The bathtub carrier can also be tilted up for feeding, and most importantly, allow others to be close without the risk of injury.

Always think before you handle an infant with severe OI. Maximize full body support with fingers spread wide, and minimize the amount of handling by using special carriers.

Feeding

Many babies with severe OI are reluctant or slow eaters. As with all infants, if they can and will suck, encouraging the nipple is important. Parents can help with feedings in the hospital to maximize proper nutrition. Tube feeding is another feeding alternative which, obviously, will not encourage the sucking instinct.

Weak muscles sometimes make eliminating gas and waste difficult. Often the build up of gas, rather than broken bones, contributes more to infant distress. Burping a child with severe OI can be difficult. Fractures may prohibit lifting, bouncing, or patting on the back to relieve an air bubble. If possible, with the baby lying on her back on a waist-high surface, lean forward until your shoulder barely touches the baby, support the infant securely, and position him or her on your shoulder while leaning backwards. Then take gentle bouncing steps and rub the back gently. Consult your pediatrician concerning products to relieve feeding or elimination problems.

Therapy and Infant Stimulation

At first, stimulation will be ever so gentle. Music, soft touch, stroking, singing, and talking are very important. Many babies will not tolerate loud or sudden noises. Startling an infant with OI can either aggravate current fractures or lead to new ones.

As soon as the infant will tolerate handling, a bath will be in order. A bath can be a great place to encourage movement. While supporting the baby's head, the baby can float, twist, turn and kick. Remember to have all bath supplies within reach before beginning a bath. Organization and planning ahead will be necessary for many tasks when caring for your baby. Businesses call it "risk management" and for you, it will become a part of your life every minute.

Balancing a risk free environment with the mental, physical and emotional stimulation your baby needs, will be challenging. You will gradually learn how to test for tolerance without hurting your baby.

Being a Parent of a Newborn with Severe OI

One parent was told to "just get back to normal" as they left the hospital with their week-old child. The anger at that statement lasted almost two years. For this family, eventually life settled; not back to normal, for there was no going back for them, but rather the established a new way, a new road. These parents realized that expecting things to return to the way they were prior to the birth of their child with OI was unreasonable, but that striving for their own interpretation of "normalcy" was the healthy thing to do.

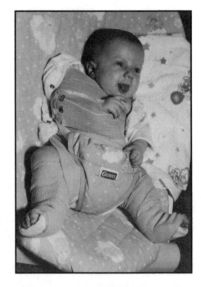

Parents eventually learn that their child's OI, no matter how all-encompassing it may initially appear, is really only a small part of who their child actually is. In most ways, they learn that their baby is like any other. The limitations of OI will eventually become insignificant, as people focus more on whole child and less on the OI.

Initially it is you, the parents, and usually the mom, who has a handicap. You are the one who must adapt to the limitations of where you go, when you go, how you go, what you can get done, etc. Your handicap came all at once, as a shock and surprise, much like an auto accident. As your child grows, the handicap will become more theirs and less yours. From experience you will learn to cope with your handicap. Your example will demonstrate to your child how to cope with his or hers.

It becomes extremely important to balance the needs of yourself, your spouse, your other children, and the child with OI. No, you probably will not be perfect at it, no busy parent is, even under ideal circumstances. The right balance will be what is comfortable for you all. One parent of a child with a severe heart condition concluded that for her own self-fulfillment she needed to be with, and care for her child. For her, getting away was not relaxing or fulfilling. Each parent will be different. Just be honest with yourself and don't expect to be the "super parent" because you have a child with OI. You will get very good at preventing accidents, but you will probably not be able to obstruct them all. Try to minimize but accept accidents and fractures and go on. Just do your best, no guilt.

Most likely the first few weeks of your baby's life will be one of the periods of greatest change in your life. Robert Marion, M.D., a pediatrician and geneticist in New York has written a book called "The Boy Who Felt No Pain". The author tells true stories of special children and the invaluable lessons they taught him. In one story about a little girl, he recounts a vivid lesson about the changes parents of children with disabilities must endure. He had just viewed a video of a couple made weeks before the birth of their daughter.[1]

"I was held spellbound by that documentary. It drove home to me the fact that the people who come to my office, the parents of children who have been born with some congenital malformation or syndrome, are not the same people they were prior to the birth of that child."

Parents of children with OI become different people. Fortunately, much of their transformation, when viewed from a distance, is generally positive, educational, and uplifting.

Works Cited

Dubowski, Frances M., R.N. and Glauser, Heidi, *"The Care of a Baby and Child with Osteogenesis Imperfecta"*, *The Osteogenesis Imperfecta Foundation, Inc., 1986.*
Routburg, Marcia, *"On Becoming a Special Parent"*, *Parent Professional Publications, 1987.*
Dickman, Irving, and Gordon, Sol, M.D., *"One Miracle at a Time"*, *Simon and Schuster, 1985.*

Endnotes
1. **Marion, Robert M.D.**, *"The Boy Who Felt No Pain"*, *Addison-Wesley, 1990, pg 31.*

Chapter 22

Suggested Techniques for Handling the Infant or Child with OI

by Heidi C. Glauser
Pittsburgh, Pennsylvania

Because the bones of infants and children with OI can fracture very easily, caregivers must take extra precautions when and handling them. All handling should be undertaken with slow, methodical movements. During periods when the infant is healing from a fracture, it is especially important to think ahead and plan the next step in the care process. For example, before lifting an infant with OI, plan where you will place her, eliminating the need for more handling than necessary.

Young Infant being Lifted

Lift and carry an infant with OI using very slow and methodical movements. Before the baby achieves head control, lift by placing one hand behind the head and the other under the

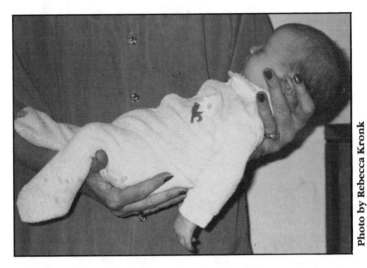

Photo by Rebecca Kronk

buttocks. Always assure that the legs and arms are not caught even slightly in a blanket or other object as you lift. If a fracture exists, it is best to use a foam pad or other flat support under the infant, thus providing even support of all limbs and minimal movement of the fractured bone.

Infant or Child with Adequate Head Control Being Carried

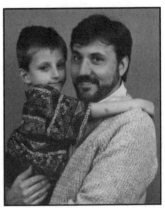

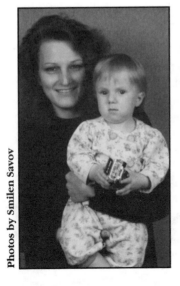

Photos by Smilen Savov

As head control develops, the child can be carried facing forward or towards the caregiver. Support the child under the crotch and around the torso, being especially careful not to apply too much pressure on the ribs.

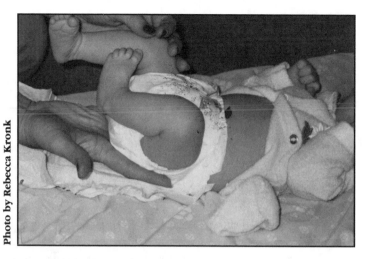

Photo by Rebecca Kronk

Changing a Diaper

Avoid holding the baby by the ankles when changing a diaper. With a flat hand first slide the clean diaper under the soiled one, unfasten the soiled diaper, and gently pull it from under the baby. After cleaning the baby, the fresh diaper, which remains, can then be fastened. When painful fractures prohibit even slight movements, some parents eliminate frequent diaper changing by inserting sanitary napkins inside the diaper and then replacing them as necessary.

Turning an Infant When a Fracture Exists

Sometimes fractures make it difficult to turn an infant from front to back. Parents have found that two people can safely and painlessly turn a small baby using the "double foam method". Prepare two flat

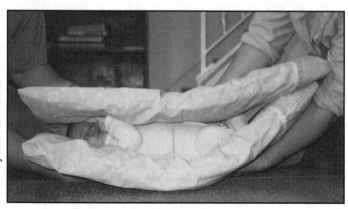

Photo by Rebecca Kronk

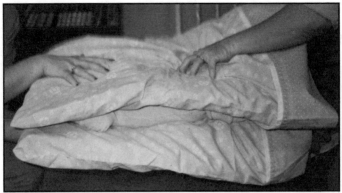

pieces of high density foam cut to a size slightly larger than the infant. The foam should be covered with pillowcases or other absorbent fabric. When a fracture occurs, place the infant on one of these foam cushions. Turn the infant's head to one side. Lay the second cushion on top of the baby, so she is "sandwiched" between the two. To turn the baby, one person stands at the baby's head and the other at the feet. Four hands are placed outside the foam cushions. Person 'A' would put her right hand and person 'B' her left hand on top of the cushion. The remaining two hands support the infant under the foam. Both people must agree in advance on the direction the baby will be turned. On the count of three, the caregivers both gently squeeze hands together, lift, and turn both foam cushions and the baby in one motion. The baby's position is painlessly changed, the top foam is removed, and a clean covering can replace the used one for the next time.

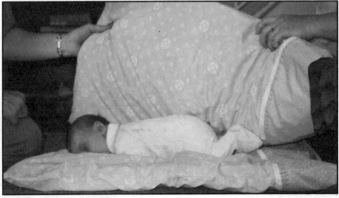

Chapter 23

Bones, Fractures, and First Aid Treatment

**By Heidi C. Glauser, Pittsburgh, Pennsylvania
and Sue Phillips, R.N., Urbana, Illinois**

What is bone?

Our skeletons make up the framework of our bodies. The bones serve as the scaffolding to protect vital organs and to facilitate movement. There are about 206 bones in the adult body. One quarter of bone composition is water, another quarter is collagen fibers, and the remaining half consists of calcium, phosphorus and other minerals.

How do bones grow?

We know that they grow in three ways:
- Bones grow in length during childhood by adding new bone at the growth plates which are located at the ends of the bones.
- Bones grow in thickness by depositing thin layers of bone on

their outside surfaces, much like the trunk of a tree.

- Bones constantly remodel or tear down and rebuild themselves in order to shape themselves and to respond to stress.[1]

How do the bones of people with OI fracture?

Bones fracture in different ways. The long bones of the body, such as the femur, or thigh bone, break differently than the more compacted vertebrae. Every time a person moves, stress is placed upon the bones by both gravity and muscle. Especially in very young children with OI, bones can fracture simply from the involuntary pull of a muscle. In all people, if the stress upon the bone exceeds the bone's internal strength and the muscles are not strong or bulky enough to protect it, a fracture can occur.

With OI, most fractures that require treatment involve the long bones. Fractures of the skull and pelvis do occur, but usually only as a result of significant trauma.

Curvature or deformity of the bone adds to the likelihood of fractures. This theory can be tested by pressing the tip of a straight finger down onto a hard surface. Notice how much pressure can be exerted onto the straight column. Now try it again, but this time, bend the finger into a "C" shape and press down. Notice the limited amount of weight the curved shaft can sustain? A similar experiment can be tried using a straight and a bent drinking straw. The result is the same. The degree of curvature in bone can dramatically affect the likelihood of fractures.

Is there anything a person with OI can do to prevent fractures?

Exercise, muscles, and weight-bearing play important roles in decreasing the fracture rate of people with OI. In fact, regular, vigorous exercise is the only known, natural method of building bone. Sedentary people have markedly less muscle mass. They gradually exert less physical effort for shorter periods, and as they do so, the muscle mass becomes smaller, and the bones become weaker and thinner. A bone that is surrounded by strong muscle will be substantially larger and stronger than a bone surrounded by a weak muscle. Additionally, a good, solid mass of muscle acts as a protective cushion around the bone.

Weight-bearing exercises thicken bone by increasing blood flow and extra nutrients within the bone-building cells.[2] It is important to remember that weight-bearing exercises are not just limited to those that can be accomplished while standing. The arms can bear weight by pushing up from a sitting position. And with proper instruction, many people with OI can achieve weight-bearing using appropriate free weights and weight machines. Although not classified as a weight-bearing exercise, the resistance of water in swimming adds weight-bearing qualities to an exercise routine.

Terminology for Various Types of Fractures

Bones can fracture in any number of ways. People with OI and their caregivers will often hear many terms describing various types of fractures and methods of treatment as described in figures 23-1, 23-2, and 23-3.

What are the Signs and Symptoms of a Broken Bone?

People with OI and their caregivers recognize a fracture in many different ways. What follows is a list of symptoms reported by people with OI. At the time of a fractures, a person may recognize only a few of these symptoms, many, or none at all:

- The person hears or feels the break
- Extreme pain is experienced
- Pain is felt when trying to use the injured body part
- The injured area swells and/or appears blue
- The injured body part hurts when touched or moved
- The injured limb appears deformed or different or moves differently than before
- The injured limb or body part is difficult to move. (It is important to note that ease of movement does not rule out the possibility of a fracture.)
- Nausea
- Vertebral fractures can lead to a loss of continence or tingling in the limbs due to nerve compression.
- The injured area feels better after being wrapped in an elastic bandage.
- In children, they cry out in a sudden, high-pitched voice, ("the broken bone cry,") at the time of injury.

Fig. 23-1	Types of Fractures
Compression fracture Occur often in vertebrae. May develop as a result of jarring. Compression fractures are often wedged, so that the front of the vertebrae is compressed more than the back. Contributes to spinal deformity.	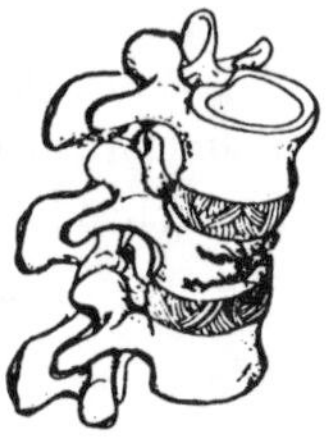
Comminuted fracture A fracture in which the bone is splintered into several pieces. Usually occurs in car accidents or when rapid force is applied to the bone.	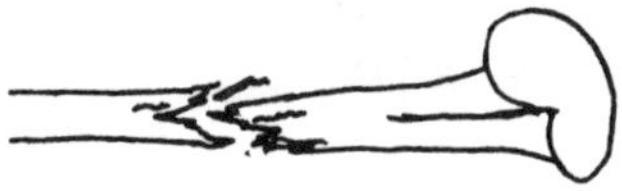
Incomplete or Greenstick fracture When the bone does not break all the way through. Common in the long bones. The term "greenstick" comes from the appearance of the fracture resembling a partly broken tree branch.	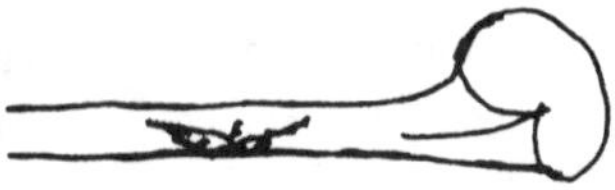

Artwork by Brian Young

Fig. 23-2	**Types of Fractures**
Complete Displaced fracture When the crack in the bone goes all the way through the bone and the pieces of the bone separate.	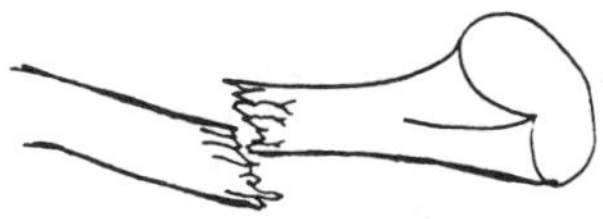
Complete Undisplaced fracture When the crack in the bone goes all the way through the bone. The pieces of the bone do not separate.	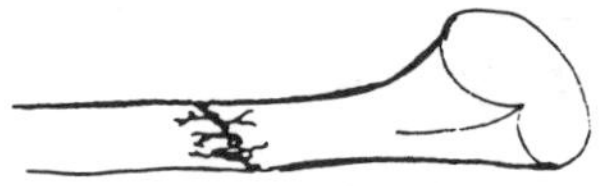
Impacted fracture When the one piece of the fractured bone is pushed down upon the other piece.	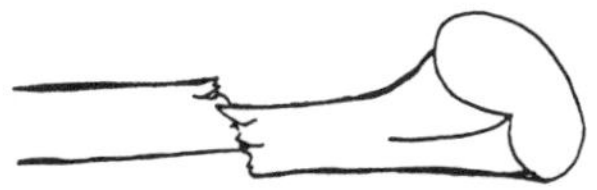
Angulated fracture When the two pieces of the fractured bone rest at an abnormal angle.	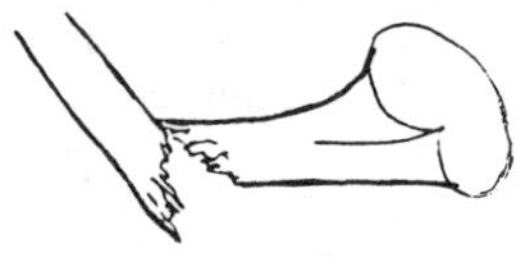

Artwork by Brian Young

Fig. 23-3	Types of Fractures
Microfractures When small parts of the bone fracture. Often these tiny fractures are not visible on X-rays. A stress fracture results when many microfractures occur and the healing process cannot keep up.	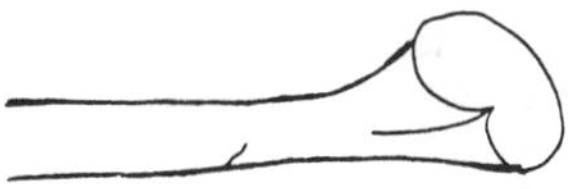
Intra-articular fracture When a fracture occurs partially or entirely within a joint.	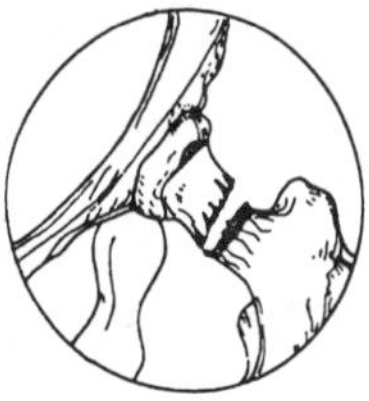
Open or Compound fracture When a fractured bone protrudes through the skin. **Note:** In the more severe types of OI, compound fractures rarely occur since the bone generally lacks the rigidity necessary to protrude through the skin.	

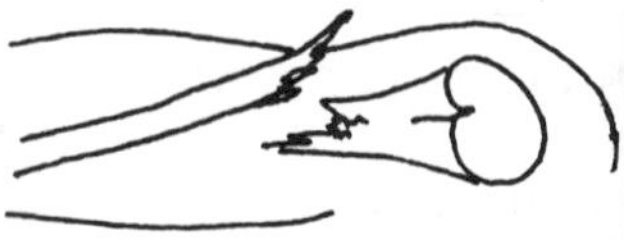

Artwork by Brian Young

What Should I Do When a Fracture Occurs?

When a fracture occurs, it is most important to stay calm and make any and all movements as gently as possible. Remember that generally the treatment of a fracture does not require immediate action. It is often best to wait until everyone involved is calm before proceeding with treatment. Help make the person with the fracture as comfortable as possible and administer pain medication if necessary. If another person was involved in the cause of the fracture, try to assure them also. Usually, when people with OI sustain a fracture it is the fault of no one, yet extreme feelings of remorse and guilt can occur.

What Extra Precautions are Needed for an Open Fracture?

If an open fracture has been sustained, additional precautions must be taken. Never attempt to push rods or bones that are protruding from the skin back into the limb. Only an experienced physician should try to set a fracture or push bones or rods back into place. Sometimes when an injured limb is splinted, the bone may slip into the correct position on its own. Never wash or insert medication, your fingers, bone fragments or anything else into open fracture. It is also important to not offer the person anything to eat or drink right after an open fracture.

First Aid for Fractures - Splinting

Much of the pain associated with a fracture occurs when the broken bone is moved. Splinting can be used as a temporary method of immobilization prior to receiving medical treatment. Also, splinting is a means to provide relief from pain and allow healing when the person with OI or caregiver determines that the fracture is not severe enough to warrant medical attention. The main goal of splinting is to provide comfort and support to an injured body part and to make transporting that person safer and easier.

Splints may be rigid such as those made from metal, plaster or wood, or flexible, and made of materials such as felt, heavy paper, or leather. Examples of some items that have proven to be effective splints by people with OI and their families include:

- a magazine
- newspaper
- elastic or Ace bandage
- towel

- air splint
- vacuum splint (conforms converting from soft to rigid in seconds)

- broom handle
- straight stick
- a flat board
- a table leaf
- corrugated cardboard formed into a three-sided tube
- rolled up blankets and towel
- an umbrella
- a brace or orthopedic device used previously by same person

- mailing tube
- "popsicle" sticks
- oatmeal box
- plaster or casting material
- a commercial splint
- padding between the legs, and strapping or tying a broken leg to the other leg
- binding an injured arm to the torso

How is a Splint Applied?

The technique chosen for splinting depends on the size of the person with the fracture and the reason for the

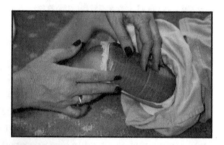

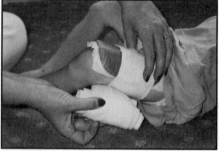

Photos by Trevor Gauser

splint. All splints should be padded with clean soft cloth, cotton, towels, or linens. The splint should extend past the joints on both sides of the suspected fracture site. When using a board to

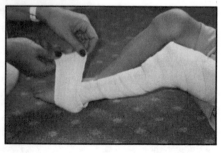

splint, be especially careful to pad it well with fabric or towels. Make sure the ends of the board extend well beyond the body part you are splinting.

Splints can be tied in place with strips of clean cloth, handkerchiefs, neckties, rope, an elastic bandage or tape. Never tie a splint on so tightly that circulation is impaired. If the person reports numbness or tingling or is unable to wiggle fingers or toes after the splint is in place, loosen the tie to prevent nerve damage or restricted circulation. Proper circulation is assured if fingernails or toenails are normal fleshy color, and do not have a bluish tint.

After applying a splint check the person's toes and fingers frequently for swelling, color changes, and pulse. If the splint cuts off the pulse or causes other problems such as, numbness, bluish discoloration, or increased swelling, loosen it or remove and reapply it more loosely. Instructions are given in figures 23-4, 23-5, and 23-6 for various methods of splinting fractures.

Tips From Parents of Children with OI when Dealing with Fractures

- When traveling keep splinting supplies handy. In cases of mild OI it is especially important to take along a physician's letter stating that the child has OI to avoid any false accusation of child abuse. Be prepared!
- Keep a frequent check on color, temperature, and blood circulation to the injured body part. Report any changes or concerns to your doctor.
- Elevation of the fractured part above the level of the heart and the application of ice will aid in comfort and decrease the amount of swelling. Some parents use bags of frozen vegetables as cold compacts since they are generally handy and malleable.
- To increase the child's level of comfort during fracture treatment, bring a favorite toy, blanket, or book.
- Stay calm and use slow, gentle movements. This is difficult when the person is in pain, but it is very important.
- Remember that dealing with fractures becomes easier for caregivers and for the person with OI as they both gain experience.

Fig. 23-4	Methods of Splinting Fractures
Splinting the Wrist or Forearm	Gently bend the fractured arm at the elbow and place the forearm across the person's chest. With the palm on the chest and the thumb pointing towards the chin, place a padded splint on either side of the forearm or wrap it with folded newspaper. The splint should extend from the elbow to the hand, beyond the wrist. Tie or tape the splint in place both above and below the fracture site. Support the splinted forearm with a wide sling tied around the neck. While resting in the sling the fingers should be about 3 inches higher than the elbow.
Splinting the Elbow	Elbow injuries may involve circulation difficulties. Do not change the position of the elbow. If the elbow was broken while straight, do not try to bend it to put it in a sling. And vice- versa, if the elbow is bent, do not straighten it. Instead, pad the armpit with a cloth and pad the arm on both sides. Be sure to secure the arm using a tie or tape, above and below the fracture site. Put the arm in a sling and tie it around the neck. If possible, additional immobilization can be achieved by securing the arm in the sling to the chest with cloth. The cloth should be wrapped around the outside of the sling, and tied under the uninjured arm.
Splinting the Upper Arm	Pad the armpit with a cloth. Carefully bend the elbow to a 90 degree angle, if possible. Place the forearm across the person's body. Place a padded splint on the outside of the injured upper arm and secure it with a tie or ace-bandage, above and below the fracture site. Tie a narrow sling around the neck to support the forearm at the wrist, making sure there is no upward pressure on the fracture site. To further immobilize the fracture, use a towel, cloth, or pillow case to secure the arm to the chest. Pass this binder around the outside of the sling and around the body. Tie it under or near the uninjured arm. To help decrease pain, place the person in a sitting or semi-sitting position if possible.

Fig. 23-5	Methods of Splinting Fractures
Splinting the Clavicle (Collar Bone)	The weakest, most frequently fractured part of the clavicle is approximately one third of the way between the shoulder tip and the center of the chest. From a position behind the person, wrap an elastic bandage or narrow strip of cloth in figure eight pattern, like a harness, around the shoulders in the following manner. Bring one end of the bandage forward, under the armpit. Then pull it back over the same shoulder. Next, wrap it diagonally down across the back and under the other armpit. Come up over the other shoulder and then diagonally across the back and under the original armpit. Repeat this several times. Secure snugly, leaving enough room to slide a finger under the bandage in front of the shoulders.
Splinting the Knee	Have the person remain lying down if possible. Gently straighten the knee of the injured leg, if necessary and if it is possible to do so. Put a padded splint under the leg extending this pad from heel to buttocks. Put extra padding beneath the knee and ankle for support. Secure the splint at the ankle and just above and below the knee. Never secure a splint over the injured knee.
Splinting the Ankle or Foot	Gently take off the shoes and socks. Place the leg of the injured ankle or foot on a pillow, or folded blanket. Make sure that the pillow extends below the heel and that the edges will meet at the knee or above. Wrap the pillow around the leg. Secure the pillow in place with tie or tape. Remember to secure the splint above and below the suspected fracture site. Fold the pillow around the heel and foot as this will support the foot. Tape, tie or use an elastic bandage to secure it. Try to keep the toes visible so that you can check for proper color, temperature and circulation.

Fig. 23-6	Methods of Splinting Fractures
Splinting the Lower Leg	With the person in a sitting position or lying on their back, straighten the leg as necessary and if possible. Put a well padded splint along either side and under the leg from above the knee to below the heel. A splint that can be wrapped on three sides is often easiest to apply. Secure the splint in at least three places, being careful not to secure directly over the fracture. An alternative method is to place some kind of padding between the legs and secure both legs together. If a pillow is used for splinting, gently place it under the leg, pin the ends of the pillow together by tying or taping. Boards or broom handles can be placed on either side of the leg and secured around a pillow for extra support. Remember not to secure directly over the fracture site.
Splinting the Back	Move the person as little as possible. Send for medical help immediately. If you must move the person, keep back, neck, and head straight and in alignment at all times. This may require the aid of more than one person. A backboard or other hard surface is necessary. If possible, find something as long as the individual. Secure it around the forehead, upper chest and lower abdomen. Stay calm! All movements must be gentle, slow and concise. If the person is face down, get help to turn the person as a unit in good alignment. Keep the person warm. Place rolled up towels, blankets, or cloths around the head, neck, and trunk to immobilize and keep from shifting position. If you are transporting a person with a back injury yourself--drive very carefully and smoothly to prevent further injury.

How are Fractures Treated?

After arrival at the hospital or doctor's office, a decision will be made as to the best method of treatment for the patient. Figure 23-7 describes the various terminology used to describe treatment methods for fractures. The treatment of choice depends upon the severity and location of the fracture, the condition of the bone, and the preferences of the doctor, the patient, and the caregiver. Often, people with OI and parents of children with OI, play an important role in the decision about the best treatment method. People with OI must become advocates for themselves in assuring appropriate medical treatment. Becoming

Fig. 23-7	Treatments for Fractures
Treatment	**Description**
Reduction	Putting the two ends of the bone into a straight alignment.
Closed reduction or Setting a fracture	When the two ends of a fractured bone can be put back into alignment without an incision.
Cast	A plaster or fiberglass form used to immobilize a fractured bone.
Splint	A plaster or fiberglass form, usually applied only partially around the broken limb.
Traction	A steel pin is passed through the bone temporarily to counteract the pull of the muscles and help the bone align correctly.
Open reduction	A surgical incision is made and the fractured bone is reduced.
Internal fixation	A device such as a plate, screw, or rod is used to hold the bone pieces in good position. Used generally when open reduction is advised.

educated about OI and its treatment will work to your advantage when seeking the respect of an attending physician.

When people fracture their bones, the classical treatment method is to immobilize the fracture in a cast. Casting, however, may not always be the best way to treat a fracture. Sometimes a lightweight splint is used. A current method of treating fractures is to put pins through the bone above and below the fracture, and then to apply an external device that will completely immobilize the section of the bone without affecting the use of the affected limb. Although rather clumsy to look at, with this fixation device, it is possible to continue use of the limb since it is not immobilized. Avoiding immobilization is a great advantage for people with thin bones.[3]

How does Healing of Bone Occur?

As soon as a bone is broken, bleeding occurs at the broken ends, the surrounding tissues swell, and generally there is extreme pain. The bleeding that occurs at the fracture site is the beginning of the healing process.

Once aligned, the bone is immobilized, usually with a cast or splint. Immobilization keeps the bone in proper position and allows a clot to form at the broken ends and healing to begin. After time, the blood clot at the fracture site becomes like the consistency of gelatin, followed by formation of strands of fiber and tissue which eventually achieve the consistency of clay. This phase continues for ten to twenty-one days after the fracture occurred. During this time the fracture is still very fragile and care must be taken to keep the site immobilized. As the fracture continues to heal, a callus develops. This callus can be easily seen on an X-ray and sometimes can be felt through the skin. This process is called ossification and it is the way the body repairs a broken bone. Gradually, the callus is reabsorbed and replaced with new bone. When the pieces of bone grow completely together as they should, it is called a "mature union." It can take as long as one year before the bone resembles itself entirely as it was prior to the fracture.[4] Also, the risk of refracturing the bone is greater until a mature union occurs.

Sometimes a "fibrous union" occurs when the bone pieces hang together by scar tissue instead of mature bone. Failure to form a solid bone bridge across the fracture sight is called a "non-union." It is also possible to have a "delayed union", wherein the physician expects that union to occur but it is taking longer than expected.[5] Appropriate treatment for these types of complications must be determined on a case by case basis.

Summary

Many people with OI and their caregivers fast become experts at first aid and fracture care. We hope this additional information about bones, fractures, prevention, terminology, symptoms, first aid, methods of treatment, and the bone healing process, will add to the previous levels of expertise experienced by the population with the highest level of firsthand knowledge about fractures - people with osteogenesis imperfecta.

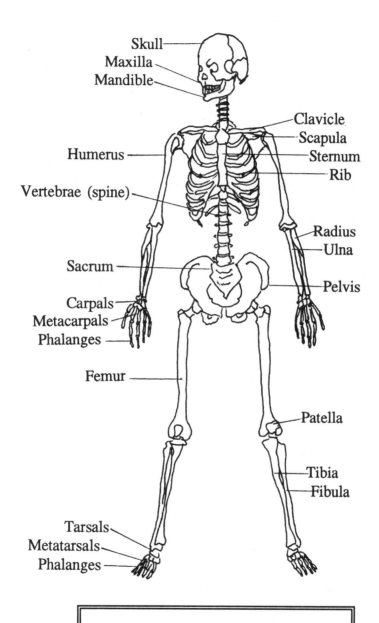

Skull
Maxilla
Mandible
Clavicle
Scapula
Sternum
Rib
Humerus
Vertebrae (spine)
Radius
Ulna
Sacrum
Pelvis
Carpals
Metacarpals
Phalanges
Femur
Patella
Tibia
Fibula
Tarsals
Metatarsals
Phalanges

Figure 23-8 **The Human Skeleton**

Works Cited

Anderson, K.N., Anderson, L.E., Glanze, W.D., *(eds.), Mosby's Medical, Nursing and Allied Health Dictionary, 4th ed., 1994.*

First Aid, The American Red Cross, 1991.

Fuentes, R., *The Family First Aid Guide, Berkley Books, New York, 1994.*

Personal Communication, Information shared by experienced parents of children with OI, March 1994.

Thompson, J.M., McFaland, G.K., Hirsch, J., Tucker, S.M., *"C.V. Mosby Co., Pocket Nurse Guide—Basic Skills and Procedures", Perry-Potter, 1986.*

Endnotes

1. **Fardon, D.F.**, *Osteoporosis - Your Head Start on the Prevention of Brittle Bones, MacMillan Publishing Company, New York, 1985.*

2. **Jacobowitz, R. S.**, *150 Most-asked Questions about Osteoporosis, Hearst Books, New York, 1993.*

3. **Bullough, P.**, *Hospital for Special Surgery, NY, (personal communication, Osteogenesis Imperfecta Foundation National Conference, San Antonio, 1992.)*

4. **Fardon, D.F.**, *ibid.*

5. **Fardon, D.F.**, *ibid.*

Chapter 24

Care of Your Fracture and Cast

by Danny K. Corbitt, M.D.
HCA Lesisville Memorial Hospital
Lewisville, Texas

Correct immobilization is essential to proper healing of fractures, sprains, and strains of the bones, joints, and ligaments. Each year, about three million people have an injury which requires immobilization with a cast. In spite of its inconvenience and discomfort, the cast helps the body heal. Healing is actually a series of events which take place over time. How fast a fracture will heal depends on many things such as the age and general health of the person, the type and location of the fracture, medications the individual may be taking, and other factors.

Types of Casts and Their Care

Generally, casts are made from either plaster or fiberglass. Plaster is the most common and traditional cast material. It is generally used in the acute stage of fracture healing because it is easily molded to the contour desired by the physician to hold the fracture in the correct position.

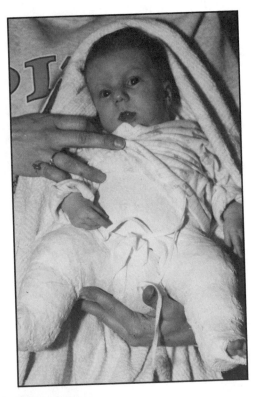

Plaster of paris contained in gauze strips or rolls is activated to a crystal form by soaking the gauze in water. The strips are then layered and formed into the proper shape. Hardening begins in five to ten minutes. However,

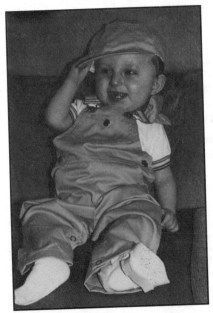

underlying layers do not harden completely for two to three days. During this time, the person must avoid putting weight on the cast or resting it on a hard surface which might cause the underlying layers to dent or shift in formation. Doing so might cause a pressure area against the skin, resulting in a sore.

Plaster casts can not be allowed to get wet. They will slowly become soft, and the correct position of the fracture could be lost. If the cast becomes wet, notify your doctor and have a new cast applied. Cover the cast with a plastic bag during bathing and activities around water to prevent it from becoming wet.

A newer form of casting material, synthetic fiberglass is lighter, stronger and more water resistant than plaster. Synthetic fiberglass casts can develop rough edges on the outside which can be lightly sanded with an emery board until smooth. If the cast becomes wet, the cast itself will not change form. However, the padding and lining beneath it will remain wet and will irritate the skin. If the fiberglass cast becomes wet, the person must take the time to dry it completely to avoid serious skin problems. Use a hairdryer set on cool to blow air under the cast until the padding is completely dry.

When a fiberglass cast is used in conjunction with the new GORE-TEX Cast Liner, the person can then participate in activities involving water. The individual may now bath regularly, wash the fiberglass cast, swim, and undergo hydrotherapy without covering the cast. The GORE-TEX Cast Liner contains billions of tiny pores that stop the passage of liquid water, but allow water vapor to pass through. Water does not wet the liner, only the skin. No special drying procedures are necessary after wetting and most patients report that the cast feels relatively dry within one hour.

Heed the Seven Warning Signs

These signs can mean that the cast is too tight, or that there is a pressure spot which could cause a sore. If any of these signs are noticed, they should be reported to the physician.

1. Extreme pain beyond the limits of the medication prescribed by the physician. It is normal to have pain at first and when the area is bumped, jostled, or

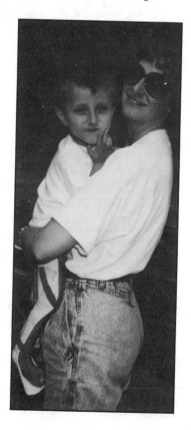

used excessively. However, pain unrelieved by moderate use of pain medicines should be reported to the doctor.

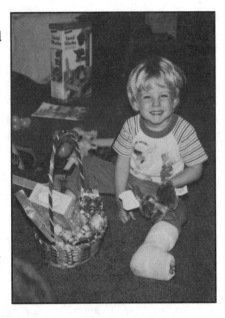

2. The cast feels too tight, and the feeling does not improve after 15 to 30 minutes of elevating the extremity above the level of the heart.

3. Persistent numbness or tingling in the extremity that does not go away after 15 to 30 minutes of elevating the extremity above the level of your heart.

4. Pain in one point under the cast that is not relieved by changing positions. This may indicate a point of pressure against the skin which could cause a sore.

5. Coldness of the extremity with a white to blue discoloration of the fingers or toes may indicate that the cast is too tight and is hindering circulation.

6. The extremity continues to swell. It is normal for the extremity to swell at first when the arm or leg is hanging down in a dependent position. Elevating it above the level of the heart allows gravity to help the fluids drain out of the extremity and back into circulation. If elevation does not help and the cast feels tight, consult the physician.

7. Any breakage or destruction of the cast.

Do's and Don'ts

Do elevate your extremity during the first few days after injury. Elevation helps reduce swelling and discomfort. Also, it may help to apply an ice-pack to the injured area.

Do exercise your fingers and toes. Exercise helps reduce swelling and allows earlier function after the cast is removed.

Don't use objects to scratch underneath the cast. You can cause serious damage, and objects lost beneath the cast can lead to pressure sores, abrasions, and even infections.

Don't ever attempt to remove the cast yourself. Removal should always be done under the supervision of your physician.

Do use a hairdryer set to coolest position to decrease itching. Blow the cool air into the end of the cast.

Do use a small amount of talcum powder to ease itching.

Cast Removal

The physician uses a special saw to remove your cast. Its blade vibrates back and forth rather than turning in a circle, protecting you from accidentally being cut. Removal of a cast should be painless and relatively quick. To help children who are frightened by the noise of the saw, some parents provide earplugs or a portable tape player for their child during the cast removal procedure.

When a cast is removed, you will notice several things.

1. The extremity may seem smaller, thinner and weaker than before the injury. This is due to a shrinking of the muscles, called atrophy, and is caused by not using the muscles while the extremity was in the cast. Through proper physical therapy and use of the extremity as directed by the doctor, muscle size and tone can usually be restored.

2. The skin will be thick and scaly in appearance. Layers of dead skin and hair, which would normally have washed off daily, have not been removed while the cast was in place. Your skin may also be over-sensitive to touch, and the normal sweat pattern may be changed. The scaly build-up on the skin will come off quickly with bathing and use of mild skin lotion. The other changes are temporary, and the skin will return to normal over time.

3. There may continue to be swelling of the injured extremity for several weeks or months after the injury. While bothersome, this is normal. Elevate the extremity whenever possible and try to avoid tight clothing which could further reduce the flow of fluids out of the extremity.

Resume Activities Slowly

It is customary that the cast will be removed before your body has completed the fracture remodeling phase of healing. When you resume your normal activities, whether work or play, do not exceed the recommendations of your doctor and therapist. When you work as a partner with your medical team, you have the best chance of healing properly and regaining normal bone and muscle strength.

Chapter 25

Physical Activity and Exercise Guidelines for Persons with OI

by Ronald Adams
Director of Recreational Therapy and Adaptive Physical Education
Kluge Children's Rehabilitation Center
University of Virginia Medical Center, Charlottesville, Virgina

It is natural for people with OI and parents of children with OI to be concerned about engaging in active exercise. The purpose of this discussion is to emphasize the importance and appropriateness of activities with the goal of improving overall health, mobility, and socialization.

Since most fractures result from trauma and falls, it is understandable why attention has focused on restrictions of physical activity. Although reasonable caution has not been abandoned, most medical authorities contend that such restrictions are no longer appropriate and are actually harmful for many people with OI.

The wide variations in the level of severity of OI must be considered for each individual prior to their involvement in general exercise programs. In this work, those with severe levels are defined as having a history of multiple fractures with marked deformities of the limbs, are short-statured, and generally use wheelchairs for their primary means of mobility. Those with moderate levels have experienced more lower-limb fractures with some experiencing delayed growth. Most are competent ambulators, with some requiring a cane or crutches for support. Individuals

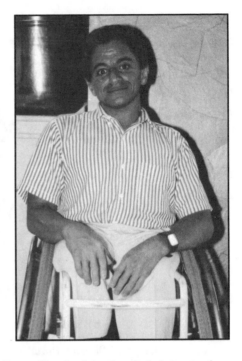

with milder OI are generally capable of independent ambulation, and have occasional fractures, few fractures, and near-normal height.

Exercise Considerations

Evidence supports the fact that a well-balanced physical activity program promotes musculoskeletal benefits and regular exercise offers a degree of protection from osteoporosis. Therefore, persons with OI should maintain as high a level of activity as possible in their daily lives. They should begin at an early age for the most physical benefit and strive to achieve a healthy sense of competence. Of course, prior to embarking on any exercise program persons with OI should consult with their doctor.

Sports Participation Guidelines

The Academy of Orthopedic Surgeons has designed participation guidelines for common physical disability groups including OI. These guidelines take into consideration the risks inherent in various sports. The information is designed to serve as a general guideline only. As mentioned earlier, exceptions may apply according to each individual case. Figure 25-1 shows ratings of sports in the following categories:

R - Recommended sports in which most individuals with OI can participate safely.

I - Individualized activities in which an activity is inappropriate for some people with OI, but may be possible for others who have less physical involvement.

X - Contraindicated sports, in which the risks outweigh the benefits for all persons with OI

Figure 25-1	Sports Participation for OI[1]		
R - Recommended for most people with OI			
I - Individualized according to the person with OI			
X - Risks outweigh benefits for all people with OI			
R	Archery	I	Bicycling
R	Tricycling	R	Bowling
R	Canoeing	I	Diving
R	Fencing	R	Field events
R	Fishing	I	Golf
I	Horseback riding	R	Rifle shooting
R	Sailing	I	Scuba diving
I	Skating (roller & ice)	I	Skiing (downhill)
R	Skiing (cross-country)	R	Swimming
R	Table tennis	R	Tennis
R	Tennis (wheelchair)	R	Track
R	Track (wheelchair)	I	Weight lifting
R	Wheelchair poling	I	Baseball
I	Softball	I	Basketball
R	Basketball (wheelchair)	X	Football (tackle)
I	Football (touch)	I	Football (wheelchair)
X	Ice hockey	X	Sledge hockey
R	Soccer	I	Volleyball

Exercise and Activities for Persons with Mild or Moderate OI

For persons with OI who are moderately affected, recommendations about participation in active exercise are often based on the clinical history of previous fractures. Additionally, restricted lower-extremity function causes difficulty in engaging in many of the traditional team sports unless appropriate adaptations are made.

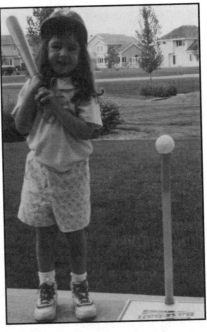

Suggested non-weight bearing activities, in addition to swimming, include stationary cycling, mat exercises, and weight training. Those activities are designed to maintain or increase strength and flexibility. Physicians usually agree that weight training with light resistance is safe. Specific skeletal sites can be isolated for strengthening using free weights and/or resistance equipment. Weight training should be done from a sitting or supine position. The participant must have the functional ability to stabilize the shoulder girdles and to move with resistance through the full range of motion. Workloads can slowly be increased and adherence to a regular training program is important.

Persons with mild OI can usually participate in active forms of exercise, including aerobic physical activities of relatively low resistance but with continuous prolonged movement. Such aerobic-type exercises can include brisk walking (3½ - 5 miles per hour) and long-distance cycling. Outdoor games, such as badminton and "Frisbee" are low risk and should be encouraged. Basketball is a popular sport, and many participate in free-play situations rather than in organized games. Preschool and primary-grade children should engage in motor fitness activities including supervised playground play, object relays, and ball-handling games.

Lifetime sports such as archery or tennis are highly recommended because they can become sources of social pleasure as well as physical benefit. Hyperextension stress fractures can occur during the serve motion in tennis, however, the risk is small compared to the benefits of participation. Stress fractures occur infrequently in such sports as golf and bowling.

Preventative risk measures include exclusion from body contact or high-impact sports (e.g. wrestling, football) and accelerated speed activities (e.g. skateboarding). Most physicians caution against soccer and excessive long bone loading as seen in tumbling and gymnastics. Long distance running is an exercise option, but chronic overloading can cause stress fractures especially for those with lower-extremity deformities.

Recreational Exercise and Activity Guidelines for People with Severe OI

Because of the risk of fractures, people with severe OI need to

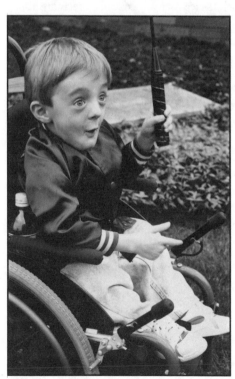

use reasonable caution, assess potential problems, and make modifications necessary to prevent injury. For example, if it is not practical to use standard swings at a public playground, parents of children with OI should consider substituting the various "risk-free" products. There are approximately 200 suppliers of adapted recreational equipment in the United States. A simple way to access these suppliers is through "Abledata", an infor-

Photo by Laura Vinchesi

mation source for adaptive equipment. (See Resource List in Appendix.)

Exploration activities teach children with OI to move effectively while learning to trust their bodies to cope with environmental changes. Such experiences can be adapted for pre-school and for primary-grade children who are not able to ambulate independently. For example, various recreational mobility aids are available, such as Hand-Karts, Hand-Cycles, Mobility Trikes, etc. Whirl-O-Wheels and Hot Wheels are popular riding toys which are appropriate due to their low center of gravity which provides exceptional stability. Safe-T-Trikes with a wide wheel base are also available. Such aides promote manual dexterity, arm strength, and eye-hand coordination.

Fishing, including pier, surf, and boat fishing, is an ideal recreational outlet for all age groups. A firm tip deep sea rod is best suited for surf fishing to reel in the line, but may present difficulty in casting, making the assistance of an able-bodied assistant usually necessary. A rod with a more flexible tip is suggested for still water fishing. Specialized equipment, such as electronically controlled reels are also available.

The Individuals with Disabilities Act, mandates that all children identified as disabled, receive physical education services. An adapted physical education program is especially important for the wheelchair user. Equipment adaptations are often necessary, including use of lightweight equipment in game situations (e.g., use a beach-ball instead of a standard volleyball). Weakness of the skeletal muscles will frequently require use of assistive devices or alternate methods to perfect a skill. For example, the use of a mobile billiard bridge mounted on two wheels

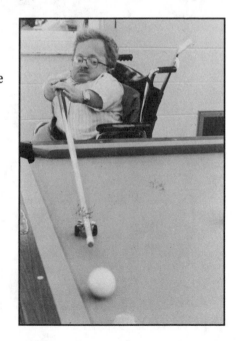

may be recommended for a billiard player who cannot balance a regular cue stick with two hands.

As stated earlier, cycling is a popular activity, and aerobic exercise can be achieved through the use of a Cyclone Wheelchair Attachment. This front wheel unit can be attached to a regular wheelchair, allowing for conversion to three-wheel mobility and handcycle propulsion. Some athletes also compete in long-distance wheelchair road racing and wheelchair basketball.

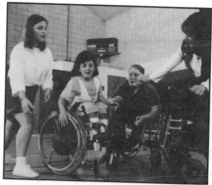

Photo by Larry Lawfer

Aerobic Fitness

Aerobic fitness programs aided in part by the many commercially available workout videotapes for private use are becoming increasingly popular. The National Handicapped Sports Organization is a leader in this field. Fitness equipment range from arm ergometers adaptable to the wheelchair user, to stair climbers for the less affected person. Stair climbers with footrests that remain parallel to the floor translate less impact loading than running and jogging, and for this reason are a popular fitness apparatus. Most people with OI need adequate time for adaptive processes to occur within the musculoskeletal system. A low to moderate intensity base needs to be established before a level of exercise tolerance is developed. The initial conditioning phase is variable depending upon each individual case, but may extend four to ten weeks, or longer.

Swimming As An Important Recreational/Therapeutic Modality

Swimming is highly recommended as it promotes joint mobility, muscle strengthening, and aerobic conditioning in a safe environment without fear of gravitational forces affecting unstable bone. If there are no medical contraindications, swimming can be started during infancy. Many swimmers with severe OI need to overcome major obstacles when learning basic skills. Because the head is the heaviest part of the body, with underdeveloped neck muscles, in many cases of OI, some beginners may require a head float. This type of buoyancy aid is popular because it provides a cushioning effect as well as support for the head. Adjustable swim rings, which encircle the neck and come in contact with less of the surface area of the head, can be used as an alternative to a head float. While a flotation device may be necessary initially, the main goal should be to swim without a support system when that is eventually possible. Physical assistance without a device is another alternative.

Buoyancy is achieved by first learning to do the back float. This is also a critical first step in learning a back stroke. When performing the supine float, an assistant can stand in the water at shoulder depth and support the beginning swimmer with one hand under the small of the back and one hand under the head. As the swimmer's balance point is found, manual assistance can be gradually eliminated as the swimmer's confidence and competence increase.

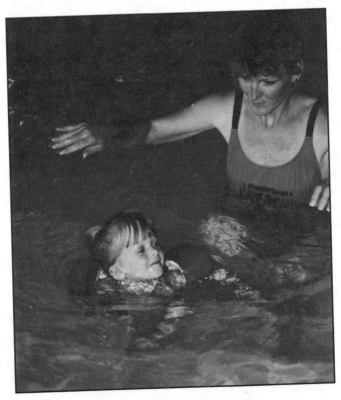

Due to limited neck mobility, some swimmers will have problems performing the breast and crawl-strokes. The back crawl and elementary back strokes are alternatives. The elementary back stroke is especially therapeutic for a swimmer with a deformed thorax. The thorax is expanded through movement of the arms, which reach diagonally upward and behind the head during the propulsive phase of the stroke, increasing lung capacity.

People with moderate OI who are ambulatory should learn the crawl stroke. This includes those who are recovering from surgery. Since weakness in the pelvic area is a common problem of OI, it is valuable to learn a flutter kick to strengthen the hip extensor muscles.

A popular swim aid is a stabilizer bar which is supported by flotation rings at each end. From the prone position, the swimmer can hold onto the bar with arms fully extended while maintaining good symmetrical alignment. An alternative to using a conventional kick-board, which is often difficult to hold onto, is a kick-board roller which has two handles attached to a plastic roller.

Post-surgical hydrotherapy for people recovering from lower-limb fractures can include gentle, active movements of the legs from the supine position. Initially the swimmer should be supported under the waist. Once weight bearing becomes feasible, it helps to have an assistant stand in front of the swimmer and provide support at waist level. Increased weight bearing is achieved through activity carried out in progressively shallower water. Waist support is gradually reduced while allowing the person to hold onto the help assistant's outstretched arms. This is eventually followed by a simple hand hold and ultimately total disengagement. Also, water aerobics and "running laps" in the pool with the aid of a flotation device are extremely beneficial for those with sufficient height to perform these exercises. The resistance obtained through water exercises adds an excellent source of muscle strengthening.

Summary

Fortunately for people with OI, there is an increased emphasis on the role of exercise in their well-being. Parents must be willing to support the interests of their child in active play at an early age and provide adaptations to physical activity when necessary. Early exercise programming often requires not only physical adaptations to the home and school environment, but also education of the parents leading to increased knowledge and decreased anxiety. All people with OI will benefit immensely from increased strength, mobility, and emotional well-being. These benefits can far outweigh the risks of potential fractures during thoughtfully planned exercise.

Acknowledgement:

A personal friend, Franz Stillfied, pictured playing billiards, contributed to the early development of this article. Franz was a dedicated public servant who advocated optimal integration of persons with disabilities into society. His active life-style and personal efforts were well recognized, especially the ongoing effort to remove architectural barriers for users of wheelchairs. Unfortunately, Franz met an untimely death due to an accident on June 20, 1988, but his valuable contributions continue to inspire me, and provide the incentive for me to continue my interest in this subject.

Works Cited

1. Proceedings of the Winter Park Seminar, "Sports and Recreational Programs for the Child and Young Adult with a Physical Disability", American Academy of Orthopaedic Surgeons, 1983.

Chapter 26

Toys and Play Things for Children with OI

**by Pat Kipperman, OTR, Omaha, Nebraska
and Jean Mandeville, Hopkins, Minnesota**

Play is an important first step in the development of all children. Through play children develop eye-hand coordination, strengthen muscles and learn basic social skills. They also begin to learn about the world around them through color and texture. Because many infants and children with OI are very small and fragile, finding appropriate play things can often be challenging.

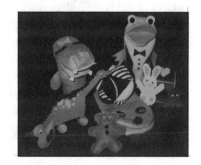

Infant Toys

Some little hands are

too small and do not have the strength to manipulate some toys. Small soft toys can be purchased or easily hand made with fabric, fiberfill, or plastic canvas. Those with bells or noise makers make fun toys that any child will enjoy. Lightweight puppets can also be fun and provide beneficial peer interaction.

Adaptive Equipment

If the child is unable to hold and manipulate toys, a free standing toy holder called a "Port-a-play" is available. This device has two plastic triangle supports with a connecting bar across the top. It is placed on either side of the child and toys can be hung from the bar to be batted or manipulated without requiring the child to actually hold them.

Switch and Battery Operated Toys

Battery operated toys and switches are available for children with very limited reach and strength. A variety of switches can be easily customized to special needs. Some of the more popular are those which turn on and off music, moving animals, and toys that make noises.

Puzzles

Puzzles with large wooden pieces are favorite play items for some toddlers, although many little ones with OI can't handle the wooden pieces. To provide a handle on each piece, small wooden beads, measuring approximately one half inch in diameter, can be securely screwed to each puzzle piece. This provides a handle on each puzzle piece so the child can easily place it in and out of the proper position.

Board Games

Board games are well-liked by many older children. For some with OI, it can be difficult to reach across a game board to manipulate the playing pieces. Plastic back scratchers make good reachers. Another alternative is to build a reacher by taking a dowel and attaching a loop of sturdy paper to the end.

Mobility Aids and Outdoor Fun

One of the greatest roads to independence and confidence is through increased mobility. The type of aid chosen depends largely on the severity of OI, muscle strength, gross motor skills, and the recommendation of the child's physician or therapist.

- Scooter boards provide mobility whereby the child lies on his stomach and uses his hands to propel himself along the floor. They can be purchased commercially or made from a padded wooden board with four large casters secured to the bottom. Carpet samples provide a comfortable padded surface on which to lay.

- Caster carts, like miniature wheelchairs, are made by attaching a small seat to a base board. Wagon wheels are secured to a rear axle and casters in the front make maneuverability simple. The child propels himself by pushing on the wagon wheels much like a wheelchair.

- A variety of riding toys appropriate for children with OI are readily available. It is important to choose a riding toy with a low center of gravity and a wide wheel base to assure stability and prevent tipping. Be sure to install a seat belt if one is not included. Some of the more popular are Hand-Karts, Hand-Cycles, Whirl-o-Wheels and Hot Wheels. Small tricycles can be adapted using wooden blocks on the pedals for short legs, and back supports for trunk stability. Some tricycles are propelled with the hands and others with conventional foot power. An alternative enjoyed by some children with OI is the Irish Mail. This has four wheels placed very low to the ground and is propelled with a pumping motion of the handlebar.

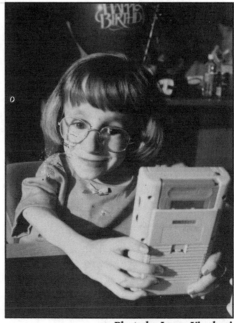

Outdoor activities become more important as the child gets older. Playground areas in parks, schools, and homes can be constructed to meet the needs of all children. One

Photo by Laura Vinchesi

example is a merry-go-round built level with the ground which would allow a child in a wheelchair to roll onto it. Chains with lock hinges secure the wheelchair and internal gears can be adjusted to allow the merry-go-round to turn at a slower speed.

Sand or water play areas can be made accessible if built onto a table, allowing a child in a wheelchair to pull up close. Other play areas can be ramped and have railings enabling use by those with braces and walkers.

Other Toy Suggestions Offered by Parents of Children with OI

Bulletin boards
Any object that makes noise
Wading pools
Magnetic toys
Felt tip pens, paints and other art supplies
Soft clay or play dough
Books
Bubble soap
Action toys, small dolls, trucks and cars
Video games

Summary

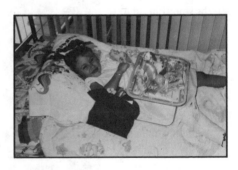

Finding toys and activities for children with OI can be challenging. Many toys are too large and heavy to be manip-ulated by those with brittle bones, limited strength, and short arms. One also has to take into consideration the lack of mobility and the need for safety. Creativity and adaptations help provide a variety of amusing playthings for children with OI.

Chapter 27

A Tailor-made Dilemma: Clothing

by Pat Kipperman, OTR
Omaha, Nebraska

The clothing that we wear can effect our physical, social, and psychological well-being. Appropriately constructed clothing can foster independence in dressing and increase the self-esteem that comes from feeling and looking good.

Every person is unique and few are blessed with perfect bodies. Features such as being short in stature, using crutches or a wheelchair, or having an asymmetrical shape can all attract attention. Right or wrong, outward appearances can often affect our opportunities for employment, promotions, and social contacts. By adjusting the fit of clothing and by selecting a stylish yet functional wardrobe, we can help others see beyond our disability to our true inner selves.

Clothing should be comfortable, attractive, fashionable, and easy to put on and take off. Specialized or adapted clothing should appear much like regular clothing. Through the use of added features and modified designs the wearer's individual needs are accommodated.

Off the Rack

For people with OI, it is sometimes difficult to locate appropriate ready-made garments. For some, petite garments or adjusted small sizes provide the perfect fit. For others it is easier to construct a garment from scratch than to modify a ready-made garment.

Sew it Yourself

For many people with OI, sewing becomes a necessary and rewarding life skill, and not just for women. Remember, many men are successful tailors.

Fabrics that allow for ample air circulation provide comfort when perspiration is a problem. Also, choosing non-cling fabrics make dressing much simpler. Natural fabrics usually are preferable to synthetics, although synthetics or blends of fiber have better wearing qualities and are often easier to maintain.

Taking accurate measurements is the secret to a good fit. Have a friend measure you in the position in which you spend most of your time. People who use wheelchairs benefit from clothing that is pleated and cut to accommodate the sitting position. When sitting, the waistline of pants and skirts tend to drop in the back and bunch up in the front. Hemlines also creep up.

Adjusting commercial patterns is relatively simple if you follow some general principles:

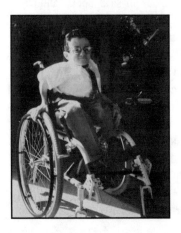

The Perfect Fit for People who Use Wheelchairs

Skirts and pants for seated people are adjusted from the crotch line to the waist. The objective is to add more fabric in the back of the pants or skirt and reduce it in the front. When you're sewing from a pattern, make three slashes, about an inch apart, on the front and back pattern pieces. These slashes should extend from the center back to about an inch from the side. Spread the back pattern piece evenly until it equals your back crotch-to-waist measurement. Overlap the front tissue until you have the desired front measurement. Use transparent tape to secure the resulting adaptation on your pattern.

When adjusting a skirt, as much fullness as possible needs to be eliminated from the back so that the wearer is not sitting on bunched-up extra fabric. The skirt should be loose around the hips and flared to fall neatly over the knees.

To adjust a jacket for the seated figure, shorten the center back panel to be even with the seat. The side panels remain the regular length. This adjustment can also be made on ready-made jackets. This does tend to look strange on a hanger, but fits very well and the difference in side length is unnoticeable while worn.

Adjustments for Spinal Curvature

To adjust for kyphosis, or "dowager's hump," slash the center back seam in the shoulder area, and spread it about two inches or more, according to the severity of the curvature. Taking a small tuck on each side of the neckline removes excess material that may form a gap in the neck area.

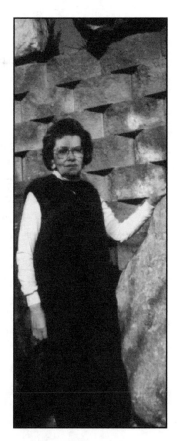

Pockets

Some people who sit frequently complain of difficulty accessing a pocket. When dressing casually, this problem can be overcome by wearing sports pants or slacks which have patch pockets placed on the thighs. Invisible zippers can be used as closures. Some people prefer pockets to be placed on the outside of the lower leg.

Crutches

People who use crutches often have a disheveled appearance caused by the movements needed to ambulate. Garments bunch up under the arms and around the crutches. Blouses or shirts can ride up making it difficult to keep them tucked in neatly. Skirt hems also become uneven. Sleeves with gussets, kimono sleeves, and raglan sleeves are very functional for crutch users as these provide extra fabric for more freedom of movement. Sleeve length may be adjusted so the sleeves do not pull up with the motion of the crutches. Blouses and shirts that are cut longer have been found to stay in place better.

Sweaters

Sweaters are a problem for many people with OI since many are hard to put on and take off. Sweaters worn by wheelchair users can bunch up around the waist and give a disheveled appearance. Hand knit sweaters offer the fit best or knitting studios will custom-knit at reasonable prices.

Underclothing

Underclothing can also present problems. Function and accessibility are very important, especially as a child starts school and wants to be independent in the bathroom. Customizing underwear can be done as follows:

- Underpants and slips can be slit down the side and closed with small snaps or Velcro.
- Many front-closure bras are available on the market, but if one's favorite brand does not offer this feature, bras can be easily converted. Sew the back closure closed. Slit the front and sew Velcro or a hook to the edges. The front may have to be extended with a small piece of seam binding to form an overlap.

Clothing for Infants

Fragile babies and toddlers with OI have different problems from those of older children and adults. Fortunately, it is easier to purchase appropriate ready-made garments for small children than adults. Clothing must be easy to take off and put on so little arms and legs can be slid into the garment without risking a fracture. In purchasing clothing, look for items that do not restrict body movements and which lie flat when opened. Sometimes buying a size or two larger than usual provides the extra room needed. Clothing should have generous neck, arm, and leg openings. Infants with OI tend to perspire excessively, making absorbent fabrics important. Many babies with OI are bothered by bright sunlight, so don't forget a sun hat when going outside. Lace, ribbons, and open-weave materials can catch small fingers and toes and should be avoided. Girls' dresses that hang from the shoulders without waistbands work very well. The top sleeve seams of shirts, blouses, and dresses can be opened and seam binding applied with small snaps. The side seam or inseam on pants can also be opened and seam binding and snaps applied to making dressing easier. As children learn to dress themselves, small pieces of Velcro can replace the snaps.

Many commercial children's patterns can be easily adapted to a flat garment by placing the shoulder seam allowances together and cutting the front and back pieces as one. This creates a wrap around garment, but can only be used with patterns that have a front closing.

Consider using a sleeping bag with a hood in place of a jacket for small infants with OI. Any measures that eliminate "dressing and undressing" have proven to be especially beneficial when little ones are most fragile.

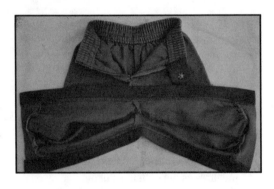

The inside leg seam of these pants has been opened and reinforced with matching fabric. Snaps or Velcro at the seam allows for ease in dressing. Also, the waist has been cut down the center-back and reinforced with a zig-zag stitch. An additional snap has been added at the waistline.

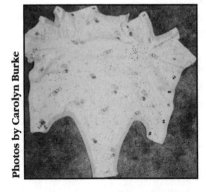

Photos by Carolyn Burke

These handy one-piece outfits have been a favorite of parents of children with OI for years. This outfit, has had the arm holes opened and snaps applied for the ultimate ease in dressing.

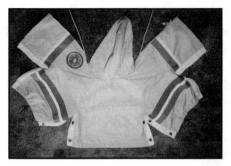

Side and arm seams on this zippered jacket have been opened and large snaps were added making cold weather dressing a cinch.

Another alternative for cold-weather dressing of a young infant with OI, is pictured here in the adaptation of this snow suit.

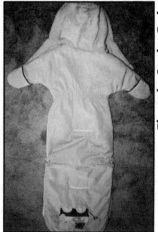

Photos by Carolyn Burke

Suggestions from Parents

- Pants with elastic waists are easier to get on and off and fit better over braces and casts.
- Polo shirts with a three-button placket allow greater arm movement when dressing.
- For smaller children, mittens without thumbs incur less risk of finger fractures as the mitten is put on.
- Remove the buttons and/or zippers from the flies of blue jeans and replace them with Velcro. Sew the button to the top of the buttonhole to camouflage the Velcro.
- Sew a "patch" to the inside of new clothing in areas where braces rub. This makes the garment last longer and gives a neater appearance.
- As a child gets older, use fabric quilt binding to encase cut edges. It is wider and stronger than regular seam binding and will wear better.
- On long-sleeve shirts, sew on the cuff buttons with elastic thread. The cuff then remains buttoned and the arms can slip right through.

Summary

By following a few simple principles, fashionable clothing that fits well and is comfortable to wear can be available to everyone. Don't be afraid to try these adaptations yourself. You may surprise yourself by discovering hidden talents. When we look and feel good, our self-confidence is increased.

Chapter 28

Adapted Equipment and Environments

by Pat Kipperman, OTR
Omaha, Nebraska

Accessibility can have a different meaning for each individual with OI. Improved accessibility can require simply arranging items for easy reach to making extensive modifications to a home. Appropriate selection and adaptation of equipment and environments can greatly enrich the life of a person with OI.

When reviewing the many available sources of information and products, follow these general principles in making selections:

- Find a reputable dealer who is knowledgeable about the product.
- Inquire as to the extent and conditions of any warranties, including initial and future service on the product.
- Do not let a salesperson talk you into a product with which you do not feel comfortable. Remember, once purchased, you must live with it every day.

Wheelchairs

New adaptations and types of wheelchairs are becoming available almost daily. The main types remain the light-weight chair and the standard heavier chair. A person with OI should take accurate body measurements prior to ordering a new wheelchair as these measurements will determine the frame size of the chair. If a wheelchair does not fit properly, its use will be limited and it may be unsafe. Choose wheelchair accessories that will increase independence and ease of movement. Preventative maintenance is also important.

- Keep your wheelchair clean by wiping it with a sudsy cloth and another cloth to dry it. Do not clean it in the shower or by using the garden hose as this can destroy the wheel bearings.
- Repair or replace worn and torn upholstery as it can become both unsightly and hazardous.
- Keep inflatable tires filled to the recommended air pressure.
- Check screws periodically to see that they are secure.

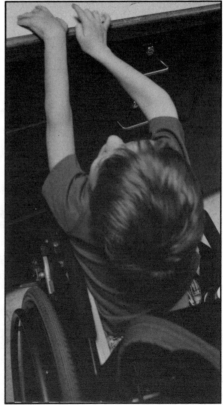

Crutches

Crutches are available in both wood and metal. Colored anodized metals are also beginning to enter the market. Crutches should be adjusted for fit while the person is in a standing position. Properly fitted, crutches should allow room to place two fingers between

Photo by Laura Vinchesi

the crutch top and the underarm. The elbow should be slightly bent. When walking with crutches, the wrist, not the underarm, should absorb the body weight. Crutch tips should be checked frequently for wear and replaced when necessary.

Walkers

Walkers also come in a variety of sizes and can be individually adjusted. When using a walker, the elbows should be slightly bent allowing appropriate leverage and safety. Wheels and tips should be checked regularly for wear and replaced to prevent slippage. Models with hand breaks on the handles provide a nice safety feature which allows simultaneous standing and reaching as the walker will stay put.

The Living Environment

Assuring an accessible home and work environment is especially important. At times, simply the physical arrangement of the environment can make a big difference in its accessibility. Also, a variety of assistive devices are available. What

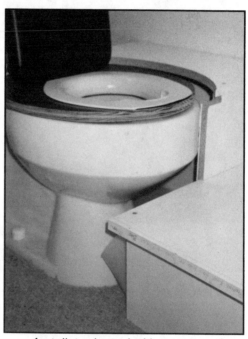

An toilet adapted with two steps for a child with OI who is capable of climbing

follows are some tips for an accessible living environment:

- Place frequently used items in places that are easily reached and those used less often on top and lowest shelves.
- Lower closet rods.
- An accessible bathroom is very important while an inaccessible one can be a dangerous area. A minimum of a 5 foot square floor area is

required for wheelchair turning and functioning.

- Grab bars in the tub or shower should be used for support instead of a soap dish handle. (The glue with which soap dishes are affixed to the wall is not sufficiently strong.) Grab bars should be installed into a wooden stud if possible. Several models fit on the edge of the tub and are excellent to take along when traveling.

- Tub/shower mats can prevent slipping and can be taken along when traveling. Getting in and out of the tub before it is filled reduces the possibility of slipping. Shower/tub bath seats or benches can be used when it is necessary to sit in the shower or tub. A hand held

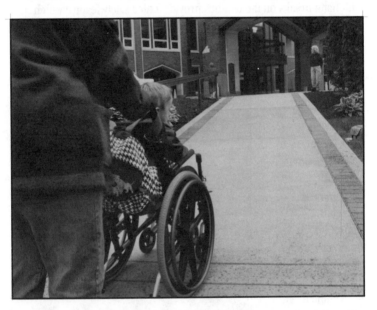

shower nozzle attached to the faucet is helpful. Some people install a temperature control in the hot water line to prevent accidental burning. Shower stalls without ledges enable a wheelchair user to roll into the stall prior to transferring to a shower bench.

- To allow optimal space for wheelchair navigation, hallways should be 42 inches and doorways 32 to 36 inches in width.

- Low pile carpeting is easier for walking and rolling wheelchairs.

- Vinyl or tile floors should not be waxed. Washing tile floors with a small amount of white vinegar in the water gives them a nice anti-skid shine.

- Switches and plugs should be within easy reach. Keep cords off the floor.

- Bi-folding or sliding doors allow easier access than standard doors.
- Scatter rugs should be removed from all areas. Bathroom carpeting is preferable in the bathroom.
- Ramps are constructed in various configurations according to the slope that is required. Several models of portable ramps are also available.

Summary

The need for adaptive equipment and environments varies widely with the OI population. Follow simple safety recommendations to reduce the chance of falls and fractures. Adaptive equipment can provide independence which will increase one's self-confidence.

Chapter 29

OI Travel - and Love It!

by Rosemarie Kasper
Hackensack, New Jersey

Many persons with OI have three major concerns when considering a travel experience: fragile bones, short stature, and hearing loss. Experience has taught strategies for dealing with them all.

Plan Ahead

Today, a variety of access guides for travelers with disabilities are on the market. Most hotel/motel directories include access information, and there are an increasing number of barrier-free facilities both in the U.S. and abroad. With appropriate planning, travelers with disabilities can expect a safe and secure journey.

Before making hotel reservations, specific and necessary information should be obtained. This might include knowing the distance from the elevator to the room; details about access to the pool area; and information about fire exits for guests with disabilities. When traveling alone, even one curb can be a monumental barrier.

When planning your itinerary, variables such as heat, altitude, and rest can make the difference between comfort and fatigue for persons with OI.

Communicate Needs

First and foremost, it is vital to communicate needs clearly to those who may provide assistance throughout the trip. These people could include a travel agent, flight attendants, hotel clerks, taxi drivers, and others who provide assistance. OI is a rare disorder — few people will be aware of our requirements.

The Specifics

When purchasing an airline ticket, specific needs such as a mobile chair to help with transportation down the airplane aisle and a request for an aisle seat should be voiced. Also, remember to mention any needs for a special diet, when reservations are made by either the travel agent or airline. Assistance needed upon disembarkation should be reconfirmed with the flight attendant during the flight.

It is equally important to convey HOW we need to be helped. For example, I explain to the flight attendants how to lift me into the aisle chair and airplane seat. It is also wise to carry a spare seat belt. More than once I've been shocked to find the tiny aisle chair did not have this safeguard!

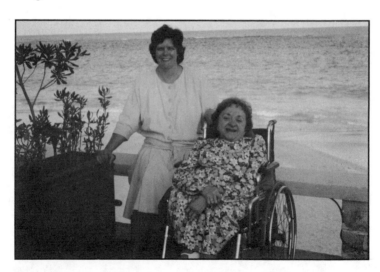

Although all new wide-body planes must have accessible lavatories, restroom facilities on most aircraft remain a major barrier to passengers with disabilities. Nonstop or direct flights are more convenient, especially, for short distances. On long flights, a stopover might be welcome, allowing time to stretch and to use the airport restroom.

Unless traveling with an able-bodied companion, a "reaching" device is indispensable on a trip. Hotel maids can be called upon to relocate towels and other needed items to be within reach. At times it may even be necessary for furniture to be re-arranged in order to access light switches or electrical outlets.

Sad but true, the Symbol of Access does not guarantee uniform accommodations. This is especially so regarding lavatories. When I travel, I always pack a screwdriver as several times my companion has removed a lavatory door, (with the manager's approval,) in order to maneuver my wheelchair through!

Cruising has recently become far more enjoyable for wheelchair users. A number of ships, including Cunard's Queen Elizabeth II, Sagafjord, and Vistafjord, and most Princess ships have specially designed staterooms for the disabled. Since it is unlikely that any cruise ship will become totally barrier-free, traveling with an able-bodied companion is recommended.

As the larger ships cannot enter certain ports of call, passengers are transferred to shore by tender, or small boat. Having endured this risky ordeal, I strongly advise avoiding it if at all possible. Since many pre-arranged tours utilize inaccessible buses, touring at ports of call may also present problems. When selecting a cruise, check whether a tender will be needed to disembark and what types of vehicles are available for sightseeing on land.

Hearing Loss and Communication Concerns

The Americans with Disability Act (ADA) mandates communication as well as mobility access. Therefore, hotels and motels are obligated to provide amplified phones or TDD's (telecommunication devices for the deaf); visual alerting devices for fire, telephone, and doorbell; and closed captioned television. The American Automobile Association (AAA) Tour Books will soon be including information on communication access in their accommodation listings.

At tourist attractions and theaters, a person who has hearing loss would benefit from asking if there is an assistive listening system. If not, copies of the text of programs or films can frequently be provided. It is also helpful to bring along a portable telephone amplifier — just in case.

Be assertive!

Most people want to be helpful but desire to know how to assist. I have obtained aid ranging from a special tour, to a ramp for the curb at our door, and a chair for the shower just by asking. Other courtesies include inviting people in wheelchairs to advance to the head of a waiting line or through a special entrance at a theater.

The Rewards of Travel

The rewards of travel are many. For me, one of the greatest has been visiting friends from Florida to California, and from Nova Scotia to Texas. A very special trip to the British Isles provided the great pleasure of visits with friends from the Brittle Bone Society in Scotland, England, and Ireland. Their supreme hospitality will never be forgotten.

I have journeyed many thousands of miles in my wheelchair by car, plane, and cruise ship. I have learned that by setting priorities, allowing time for possible delays, and taking along your sense of humor, an enjoyable journey awaits. Don't ever let OI stop you from living life to its fullest.

Chapter 30

The Osteogenesis Imperfecta Foundation, Inc.

by Gemma M. Geisman
Manchester, New Hampshire

For centuries, the challenges of living with osteogenesis imperfecta (OI) seemed insurmountable to those who had to face the prospect alone. Now, because the founders of the Osteogenesis Imperfecta Foundation (OIF) created a caring, supportive organization, the isolation has been greatly reduced though the challenges remain.

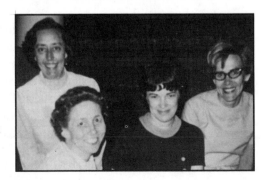

Founded in 1970 by a small group of parents, OIF is now the largest organization in the world dedicated to providing mutual support, increased awareness, education and research into the causes, treatment and cure of OI. From its modest beginnings, the Foundation has grown into a viable national voluntary health agency with a professional staff that serves thousands.

Led by a board of directors that formulates policies and oversees the financial accountability, the Foundation strives to improve the quality of life for all who have this brittle bone disorder.

Research

Applications for research grants are reviewed by a panel of scientific experts who judge the quality of the studies and their potential toward helping to unravel the mysteries of OI. The OIF Medical Advisory Council also monitors scientific advances and promotes OI research. This is accomplished through regular participation in national and international scientific symposiums on OI, often co-sponsored by OIF.

To encourage young scientists to pursue ongoing OI research under the supervision of a principal investigator, OIF established the Michael Geisman Memorial Fellowship Fund in 1981. To date, the two-year fellowship program has funded studies ranging from basic research on genetic abnormalities in collagen to using mice with OI to investigate the impact of abnormal collagen gene function on skeletal development during aging. Further, the Foundation funds seed grants, link grants, and general research grants on many OI issues. Applications for research grants continue to increase dramatically, a sure sign that the Foundation is successfully stimulating interest in the research community. Many scientists whose research projects were initially funded by OIF, have gone on to expand their studies with the support from the National Institutes of Health and other funding agencies.

To ensure the continuation of federal funding for vital research, the OI Foundation has established a Committee to Encourage Research to advocate with members of Congress and other governmental bodies. Additionally, to further the Foundation's research goals, partnerships have been formed with organizations including The Coalition of Heritable Disorders of Connective Tissues, The National Organization for Rare Disorders, The National Coalition for Osteoporosis and Related Bone Diseases, the Medical Research Agencies of America, and the Alliance of Genetic Support Groups.

Mutual Support and Education

Presenting a frank, yet positive, picture of OI to the public and ensuring that the needs of the OI Community are met are the primary concerns of the OI Advisory Council. Established to safeguard the principles upon which OIF was founded, council members are adults with OI, parents, and friends.

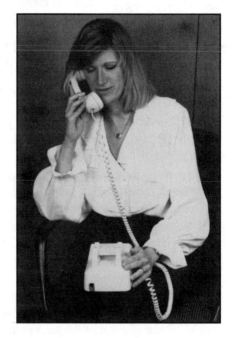

Regional managers and their teams of volunteers provide personal contact to OI families, oversee fund raising, and organize support groups that are open to all who wish to become part of the OIF family.

Breakthrough, a quarterly newsletter of the Foundation brings heartwarming success stories, problem-solving articles, medical updates, and activity and fund-raising reports to the membership. ***Backbone,*** another quarterly publication of OIF tells donors and other interested parties exactly how their funds are being used. Regional volunteer librarians distribute OIF publications, topical reprints and videos.

Periodic local and regional programs on OI are presented and, biennially, a national conference brings individuals with OI, their families, researchers, volunteers, caregivers, and support personnel together for workshops on many aspects of living with OI. These well-attended conferences create a genial atmosphere for learning and sharing experiences.

Increased Public and Professional Awareness

A Speakers' Bureau presents vital information about OI to target public and professional audiences. Videos tell the OIF story to would-be supporters and public service announcements alert television viewers about the special needs of individuals with OI.

Due to rising accusations of child abuse in undiagnosed OI, a major effort has been made by the Foundation to create professional and public awareness about this very traumatic problem that often tears innocent families apart. Targeted mailing to medical and social service agencies, news releases, and volunteers telling their stories in the media, have created publicity that must not lose momentum.

OIF Yesterday and Today – Hope for Tomorrow

In the past, parents were told that their child's fragile condition was a rarity with no known medical intervention, educational materials, or support systems available. Today, when a family member or medical professional contacts OIF for help, they are referred to a specialist or OI clinic in their area. An initial packet of literature is sent, at no charge, and information is given about area contacts and support groups. However, it is news about OI research and the hope that it brings to the parents of the newly-diagnosed which is perhaps the Foundation's greatest desire.

Recent strides in public and professional awareness of OI and in the research arena have brought much satisfaction to those who have worked continually to solve the many problems associated with OI. Yet, realistically, we know that a great deal more remains to be done. Without sacrificing its important education and support goals, the OI Foundation hopes to more aggressively pursue fund-raising and advocacy programs until the greatest challenge, a cure of OI, has been met and added to the list of accomplishments.

The hard work of many dedicated volunteers has brought the Foundation a long way. A professional staff is in place to administer the programs of the Foundation and to assist with and oversee OIF activities. But a large enthusiastic corps of volunteers is still essential to accomplishing our goals. Volunteers are involved in fund raising, advocacy, public relations, volunteer management, support services, grant writing, and general organizational development.

People no longer must face the problems of OI alone. Instead, the Osteogenesis Imperfecta Foundation offers support and contact with other families and the opportunity to join with others as a valuable member of the "striving to win" team. Perhaps someday you'll say, "Because of me, others grew stronger!"

For information on how to become involved in this Foundation, contact:

The Osteogenesis Imperfecta Foundation, Inc.
5005 W. Laurel Street, Suite 210
Tampa, Florida 33607-3836
(813) 282-1161

Appendix A

About the Authors

Ronald Adams graduated from the American University in Washington, DC where he majored in physical education. He has over 30 years of experience providing clinical recreation and physical activity services at the Pennsylvania Rehabilitation Center, Kluge Children's Rehabilitation Center where he is now employed. Mr. Adams has co-authored 4 books, published 32 professional articles, and lectured at many conferences. His interest in OI was generated through the many lessons he learned from a personal friend, now deceased, who had OI.

Peter Bullough, M.D., has been an advocate for people with OI for many years. He is a long standing member of the Osteogenesis Imperfecta Foundation Medical Advisory Council and is renowned as an speaker about OI. Along with others, Dr. Bullough established the OI Clinic at the Hospital for Special Surgery in New York City in 1970. Presently Dr. Bullough is Director of Laboratory Medicine at the Hospital for Special Surgery, and is a professor of pathology at Cornell University Medical College.

Peter H. Byers, M.D., is an internist and medical geneticist. He received his undergraduate education at Reed College, Portland, Oregon and his medical degree from Case Western Reserve University in Cleveland, Ohio. He has been at the University of Washington in Seattle since 1974 where he is now Professor and Director of the Medical Genetics Clinic. He served as the chairman of the Medical Advisory Council of the Osteogenesis Imperfecta Foundation since 1990. Dr. Byers has written numerous articles about OI that have appeared in many of the major medical and scientific journals.

David Cole, MD, Ph.D., FCCMG, FRCPC, is a biochemical geneticist at the Banting Institute, Toronto, Canada. Over the years he has become increasingly involved in the OI community both professionally and personally. He was a member of the Medical Advisory Council for the Canadian Osteogenesis Imperfecta Society, and a participant in Osteogenesis Imperfecta Foundation conferences, both nationally and internationally. His interest in the psychological and social aspects of OI stemmed from a graduate student research project he conducted along with Glenda Shea-Landry, which looked closely at the effects of OI on an individual, the family, and society at large.

Kathy B. Collins graduated from Carroll College with a BA in English and currently teaches 8th grade Middle School at Helena, Montana. She served as a Consumer Specialist through the Center for Independent Living in Berkeley, California, a board member for the Montana Independent Living Project and Rocky Mountain Easter Seals. She was named as Montana's Disabled Person of the Year in 1988 and has represented the disabled community at various state and federal hearings, including a 1992 visit to Japan.

Danny K. Corbitt, M.D., is a native Texan who graduated Summa Cum Laude with a BS degree from Texas A & M University and obtained his M.D. at the University of Texas Medical Branch at Galveston. Dr. Corbitt is a member of the AMA, the Texas Medical Association, and the Texas

Orthopaedic Association. He has been a board certified diplomat with the American Board of Orthopaedic Surgery since 1987 and a fellow with the American Academy of Orthopaedic Surgery since 1989. Dr. Corbitt practices orthopaedic surgery with a sub-specialty interest in shoulders. He is currently Chief of Staff at HCA Lewisville Memorial Hospital.

Gemma M. Geisman began her association with other parents of children with OI in 1970. After an article she wrote was published in *Redbook Magazine*, the seeds of the Osteogenesis Imperfecta Foundation were sown. The Osteogenesis Imperfecta Foundation was formed as hundreds of parents of children with OI slowly gathered to share their triumphs and tears. Ms. Geisman has worked tirelessly to build the OIF through service on numerous committees, editorship of the newsletter, Breakthrough, and as President and Executive Director. She continues today as a life member of the OIF Board of Directors.

Lynn H. Gerber, M.D., is the chief of the Department of Rehabilitation Medicine at the Clinical Center, National Institutes of Health, in Bethesda, MD. She is recognized internationally for her studies in physical rehabilitation for children with osteogenesis imperfecta. Her comprehensive rehabilitation program is designed to insure proper positioning for children with OI, promote ambulation, improve strength, and support full social and educational integration. Dr. Gerber serves on the Medical Advisory Council of the Osteogenesis Imperfecta Foundation.

Heidi C. Glauser has been an active volunteer with the Osteogenesis Imperfecta Foundation since shortly after her son was born with OI. She has served as a member of the Board of Directors since 1984, on numerous committees, and as President of the organization from 1989-1992. Ms. Glauser authored the OIF pamphlet, "Care of a Baby and Child with OI," and was instrumental in the implementation of two successful national conferences. Her experience as a leader and writer, and her broad knowledge of osteogenesis imperfecta have contributed to the editorship of this, the first book written for people and families affected by osteogenesis imperfecta.

Cheryl Greenberg, M.D., received her M.D. degree from McGill University in 1974 and subsequently completed her Pediatric Medical

Genetics specialty training at the Montreal Children's Hospital. She has been a clinical geneticist at the Winnipeg Children's Hospital since 1979 and currently is the director of the Metabolic Service in the Section of Genetics and Metabolism. Her main research interests are in connective tissue disorders. She is currently an Associate Professor in the Departments of Pediatrics and Human Genetics at the University of Manitoba in Canada.

Carole Hagin became interested in osteogenesis imperfecta when she was diagnosed with OI at age fifty. Ms. Hagin is a nurse-midwife at Kaiser Permanente medical group in Walnut Creek, California, in labor and delivery. She obtained her education as a registered nurse in 1977 and became a certified nurse-midwife in 1979. Ms. Hagin is active as a speaker at local schools and seminars, has taught numerous classes and has a manual for home birth and has authored a handbook for family centered hospital deliveries. Currently acting as preceptor for UCSF midwifery students a Kaiser, Walnut Creek, she lives in Martinez, California with her husband, Bob, and eighteen year old granddaughter, Shannon.

Rosalind James, is a past President of the Osteogenesis Imperfecta Foundation and has served as one of it's most active leaders since its inception. More recently, Ms. James role in assisting families who have been wrongfully accused of child abuse, has led her to become one of the nation's leading experts in the subject. As the mother of a college student with OI, and author of the pamphlet, "The Education of a Child with OI" her expertise in OI is broad.

Anthony Johnson, D.O., is an associate professor of Maternal-Fetal Medicine at Jefferson Medical College, Thomas Jefferson University, Philadelphia, Pennsylvania. He is currently the clinical director of the M.O.M. Center, (Making Options for Motherhood), a multi-disciplinary program designed to deliver prenatal care to women with disabilities. His specific interest in OI stemmed from his association with a young lady with type III OI whom he cared for in 1991. At 2'6" in height, her determination and eventual good fortune in successfully completing her pregnancy resulted in Dr. Johnson's initial interest in OI.

Ronald Jorgenson, D.D.S., Ph.D., specializes in research in syndrome delineations, and identification of genetic factors in oralfacial disease. Dr. Jorgenson has published papers on the dental manifestations of OI, is on the editorial boards of several journals, and is Associate Editor of the *Birth Defects Encyclopedia.*

Rosemarie Kasper is a graduate from Fairleigh Dickinson University, in Teaneck, NJ, where she obtained Masters Degree in Counseling and Guidance. She recently took retirement from her many years of service as a Senior Rehabilitation Counselor at the New Jersey Division of Vocational Service in order to devote more time to her writing. Ms. Kasper is an accomplished author with more than 100 published articles, most on disability issues. She is a past member of the Osteogenesis Imperfecta Foundation Board of Directors and she currently serves as the editor for the popular newsletter, Breakthrough.

Pat Kipperman, OTR\L., is a licensed occupational therapist, with many years of experience working with people with disabilities. She is currently the senior therapist at the Methodist Health Systems, Omaha, Nebraska. Ms. Kipperman is the author of the *Osteogenesis Imperfecta Foundation Adaptive Equipment and Reference Manual* and has served since 1993 as the Regional Manager Coordinator overseeing and providing support services for families affected by OI. Pat has OI herself and is the mother of a son with OI.

Douglas Lathrop currently serves as the vice-president of the California Chapter of the Osteogenesis Imperfecta Foundation. He is a free-lance writer whose work has appeared in a number of disability-related publications, including *Accent on Living, CAREERS* and the *disABLED.* He is currently serving as contributing editor for *Mainstream Magazine.* Mr. Lathrop has osteogenesis imperfecta and resides in Northridge, California.

Jean Mandeville, from Hopkins, Minnesota, has been actively involved in OI work since the birth of her son, Jay, in 1974. She has served as Osteogenesis Imperfecta Foundation secretary, Chairperson of three committees, and currently as President of the Osteogenesis Imperfecta Foundation. Through the years Ms. Mandeville's efforts on behalf of the OI community have been primarily in encouraging OI research.

Bradley C. McRae, Ed.D., has worked extensively in the area of stress management. Dr. McRae is the president of McRae & Associates, and gives seminars on time and stress management and negotiating skills. Additionally, he has worked with people with disabilities and their families when facing the uncertainties associated with various types of medical conditions. Participants in Dr. McRae's workshops appreciate his ability to present significant information in a humorous and resourceful manner.

Edward Millar, M.D., Orthopaedic Surgeon, and Chief of Staff, Emeritus, Shrine Hospital for Crippled Children, Chicago Unit, served as the Chairman of the Medical Advisory Board of the Osteogenesis Imperfecta Foundation for twelve years. His expertise and knowledge about all aspects of osteogenesis imperfecta is paralleled by few. Dr. Millar hosted a number of OI symposiums, co-edited a volume of *Clinical Orthopaedics and Related Research* that dealt almost exclusively with OI, and has been a committed advocate for patients with OI for years.

Rosemary Parisi, R.D., is a registered dietician at the National Institutes of Health in Bethesda, Maryland. She has held her current position at the NIH Clinical Center for 16 years and has worked directly with children with OI for the past three years. Specifically she assesses the nutritional status of children with OI and provides intervention as needed. She received her BS from the University of Tennessee and fulfilled her Dietetic Internship at Massachusetts General in Boston.

Melanie Pepin, M.S., is a certified genetic counselor. Her familiarity with OI developed while employed for ten years in the Pediatric Genetics Clinic at Children's Hospital and Medical Center in Seattle. Currently she manages the patient related service of the Connective Tissue Biopsy Program at the University of Washington in Seattle where she performs clinical research and assists with publications.

Sue Phillips, R.N., lives in Urbana, Illinois where she is a registered nurse and the mother of an 18-year-old son with osteogenesis imperfecta. Ms. Phillips received her undergraduate degree at Parkland Jr. College, and her nursing degree at the University of Illinois. She currently is employed as the nurse in the Sports Medicine Department at Carle Clinic in Urbana, Illinois.

Sandra Pinkerton, Ed.D. received her doctorate of education from Teachers College, Columbia University. She was formerly a teacher of special education and currently conducts lectures and provides consulting services in special education. She serves on the Ft. Lee, New Jersey Board of Education. Born with spina bifida, Ms. Pinkerton is a long time friend of the Osteogenesis Imperfecta Foundation.

Grace Adams Sisco is the mother of 8 year old Becky, who has OI, "best described as Type II". Grace has been active in the Osteogenesis Imperfecta Foundation as an Area Coordinator for the Intermountain West. After 6 years at home with Becky, she finished her MPA and is currently working as the Vice President of Easter Seal Society of Utah.

Peter Smith, M.D. is the attending Orthopaedic Surgeon, at Shriners Hospital, Chicago Unit. His experience in working with children with OI originated with his close work with Dr. Edward Millar, a pioneer in the orthopedic treatment of OI. Dr. Smith was a featured panelist at the national conference of the Osteogenesis Imperfecta Foundation in 1992 and has made numerous presentations and written on a number of bone related subjects.

Shannon Smith has served as an editing intern for *Living with Osteogenesis Imperfecta, A Guidebook for Families*. She has completed two years of study at Carlow College in Pittsburgh, Pennsylvania where she is a biology major. She plans to attend graduate school or medical school after graduation in 1996. Ms. Smith would like to pursue a career in the medical field.

Beth Tatman, a member of both the Osteogenesis Imperfecta Foundation and Little People of America, has studied and lectured on human sexuality for many years. She has conducted many workshops on intimacy for people with OI at the national conferences of the Osteogenesis Imperfecta Foundation. Beth, who has OI and is short statured, is proud to credit past workshop participants as the source of her expertise.

Lawrence C. Vogel, M.D. has been a pediatrician on staff at the Chicago Unit of Shriners Hospitals for Crippled Children since 1978 and has been full-time Director of Pediatrics since 1981. His interest and exposure to children and adolescents with osteogenesis imperfecta was fueled by the renowned Dr. Edward A. Millar. Dr. Vogel received his medical degree from the University of Illinois, and served his residency in Pediatrics at Yale University. His main interest is the care of children and adolescents with chronic disabilities.

Joan C. Weintrob, C.P.O., is a certified Prosthetist-Orthotist and a Registered Occupational Therapist. She is the founder and president of the Orthotic-Prosthetic Center, Inc., with offices in Fairfax, Virginia and Rockville, Maryland. Her centers provide adults and children with orthotics, prosthetics, seating systems, mobility systems, and durable medical equipment. Together with her staff of 14, she provides services to children with OI in cooperation with OI research being conducted at the National Institutes of Health.

Deborah Yarborough, an adult with OI, is a long time advocate for people with disabilities. She has served on the board of directors of the Osteogenesis Imperfecta Foundation since 1986 and as the Foundation President from 1990-1992. Ms. Yarborough worked with key legislators toward the passage of the Americans with Disabilities Act. She has authored numerous publications including, *What's True and What's Not: An Employer's Guide to Disability.* Ms. Yarborough currently works at Silicon Graphics, a 3-D visual communications company, as the Director of Diversity Programs.

Appendix B

Osteogenesis Imperfecta Organizations Worldwide

Australia
OI Society of Australia
P.O. Box 401
Epping
New South Wales, 2121
Australia

Belgium
Zelfhulpgroep OI, vzw
Meibloemstraat 12
B-9900 Eeklo
Belgium
Phone: 32-91-776727

Canada
Canadian Osteogenesis Imperfecta Society (COIS)
c/o Mary Lou Kearney, President
128 Thornhill Crescent
Chatham, Ontario
Canada N7L 4M3
Phone: 519-436-0025

Denmark
Dansk Förening för OI (DFOI)
Gøngesletten 23
DK 2950 Vedbæk
Denmark

Europe
OI Federation Europe (OIFE)
Luytelaer 1
NL 5632 BE Eindhoven
The Netherlands
Phone: +31-40-41-67-44

Finland
The Finnish OI Society (FOI)
Jouko Karanka
Rukokatu 21
SF-33340 Tampere
Finland

France
Association de l'Osteogenese Imparfaite (AOI)
76570 Sainte-Austreberthe
France
Phone: 33-35-923610

Germany
German OI Society (GOIB)
OI-Gesellschaft
Postfach 1546
63155 Mühlheim a. Main
Germany

Great Britain
Brittle Bone Society   (BBS)
112 City Road
Dundee, DD2 2PW
Scotland

Italy
Associazione Italiana Osteogenesis Imperfecta (As.It.OI)
Via Dietro Duomo 20
I 35139 Padova
Italy

The Netherlands
Vereniging Osteogenesis Imperfecta   (VOI)
Postbus 389
NL 4330 AJ Middelburg
The Netherlands

New Zealand
Brittle Bone Society of New Zealand   (BBSNZ)
c/o Mrs. Susan E. Douglas
2 Queen's Crescent
OAMARU
New Zealand

Norway
Norsk Forening for OI   (NFOI)
Postbox 114
Kjelsås
N 0411   Oslo
Norway

South Africa
South African Brittle Bone Association   (SABBA)
37 Broadway
Westville 3630
Natal
South Africa

Sweden
The OI Group of Sweden
Hannebergsgatan 22
S-17147 Solna
Sweden

Switzerland
Schweizerische Vereinigung OI (SVOI)
C/o Frau Hanne Muller
Brändistrasse 25
CH 6048 Horw
Switzerland

United States of America
Osteogenesis Imperfecta Foundation, Inc. (OIF)
5001 W. Laurel Street, Suite 210
Tampa, Florida 33607
U.S.A.
Phone: 813-282-1161

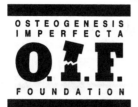

**Osteogenesis Imperfecta
Foundation, Inc.**
5005 W. Laurel St. Suite 210
Tampa, FL 33607-3836
813-282-1161
FAX 813-287-8214

National Registry Form

Reporter _____

Date _____

Relationship to patient (self/parent/physician/etc.) _____

_____

Address _____

_____

City   State   Zip

Patient Information:

Name _____

Social Security Number _____   _____   _____

Street Address _____

_____

City   State   Zip

Sex: _____ Male   _____Female

Race: _____ White   _____ Black _____Oriental _____ Other

Personal Data:

Birth Date: _____
          Month   Day   Year

Birth Place: _____
       State   Country

If Deceased, Date of Death: _____
           Month   Day   Year

Medical Information:

Delivery Type: _____Vaginal _____C-Section

Birth Weight: _____ Birth Length: _____

Fractures Present (Qty.) _____Before Birth _____During Delivery

_____After Delivery

Family members who have osteogenesis imperfecta

(Check all which apply)

_____ None _____ One Parent _____ Both Parents

_____ Sibling(s) _____ Other (Specify) _____

Diagnosed by: _____

Physician/Hospital _____

_____

| City | State | Zip | Country |

Symptoms/Conditions Experienced as of Reporting Date
(Check all which apply)

☐ Fractures throughout body
☐ Fractures mainly in arms
☐ Fractures mainly in legs
☐ Fractures in spine
☐ Sensitivity to anesthesia
☐ Blue sclerae
☐ Excess perspiration
☐ Scoliosis
☐ Loose joints
☐ More than normal bruising
☐ Anemia
☐ Other _____

☐ Short stature
☐ Hearing loss
☐ Hydrocephalus
☐ Constipation
☐ Digestive problems
☐ Teeth problems
☐ Bone deformities - bowing
☐ Heart condition
☐ Respiratory problems
☐ Hernias
☐ More than normal bleeding

(If applicable) Cause of Death _____

This national registry report will be held confidential by the Osteogenesis Imperfecta Foundation, Inc. which will use this reporting system to establish incidence and severity rates of persons with OI. Personal identifying information will not be released to researchers without the consent of the individual registering. Completed reports should be sent to the address indicated above.

OIF94PPS1

Appendix D

Additional Resources

Organizations

Adoption

Gladney Center
Maternity Home and Infant Placement Center
2300 Hemphill
Fort Worth, TX 76100
1-800-GLADNEY
1-800-922-6000 - Adoption inquiries

Aids for Independent Living

IBM National Support Center for Persons with Disabilities
PO Box 2150
Atlanta, GA 30055
Center provides information about the aid computers can offer people with vision, hearing, speech, learning, mental retardation, and mobility problems.

Child Abuse

American Humane Association
9725 E. Hampden
Denver, CO 80231

Child Abuse Listening Mediation (Calm), Inc.
PO Box 718
Santa Barbara, CA 93102

Clearinghouse on Child Abuse and Neglect Information
PO Box 1182
Washington, DC 20013

Education

American Council of Rural Special Education (ACRES)
Western Washington University
Miller Hall 359
Bellingham, WA 98225
(206) 676-3576

Council for Exceptional Children (CEC)
1920 Association Drive
Reston, VA 22091
(703) 620-3660
This Council is the largest international professional organization committed to improving educational outcomes for individuals with exceptionalities.

ERIC Clearinghouse on Disabilities and Gifted Education
Council for Exceptional Children*
1920 Association Drive
Reston, VA 22091-1589
(703) 620-3660
The ERIC Clearinghouse on Disabilities and Gifted Education gathers
and disseminates educational information on all disabilities and on
giftedness across all age levels.

Higher Education and Adult Training for People with Handicaps
(HEATH) *
HEATH Resource Center
One Dupont Circle N.W. Suite 800
Washington DC 20036-1193
1-800-544-3284
(202) 939-9320
A National Clearinghouse on Post-secondary Education for Individuals
with Disabilities, the HEATH Resource Center serves as an information
exchange about educational support services, policies, procedures,
adaptations, and opportunities on American campuses, vocational-
technical schools, adult education programs, independent living
centers, transition, and other training entities after high school.

National Association of Private Schools for Exceptional Children
(NAPSEC)
1522 K Street NW, Suite 1032
Washington, DC 20005
(202) 408-3338
NAPSEC is a nonprofit association whose mission is to promote
excellence in educational opportunities for children with disabilities by
enhancing the role of private special education as a vital component of
the nation's educational system.
National Center for Education in Maternal and Child Health
Clearinghouse*
2000 15th Street North
Arlington, VA 22201-2617
(703) 524-7802

President's Committee on Employment of People with Disabilities
1111 20th Street, NW
Washington, DC 20036-3470
(202) 653-5044
The committee's mission is to facilitate the communication, coordination, and promotion of public and private efforts to empower Americans with disabilities through employment.

General Disability Information

Administration on Developmental Disabilities*
U.S. Department of Health and Human Services
200 Independence Ave., SE
Washington, DC 20201
(202) 245-2980

Association for the Care of Children's Health (ACH)
7910 Woodmont Ave., Suite 300
Bethesda, MD 20814
(301) 654-6549

Center for Children with Chronic Illness and Disability
Division of General Pediatrics and Adolescent Health
University of Minnesota
420 Delaware Street
Minneapolis, MN 55455
(612) 626-4032
(612) 624-3939
This center is dedicated to the study and promotion of psychological and social well-being of children with chronic illness and disabilities and their families.
Publications: Children's Health Issues, Children's Health Briefs, and Springboard

Clearinghouse on Disability Information*
Office of Special Education and Rehabilitative Services (OSERS)
Room 3132
Switzer Building
330 C Street S.W.
Washington, DC 20202-2524

(202) 205-8241
(202) 205-8274
This clearinghouse responds to inquiries on a wide range of topics, particularly in the areas of Federal funding for programs serving people with disabilities, Federal legislation affecting the disability community, and Federal programs benefiting people with disabilities.

National Center for Youth with Disabilities (NCYD)
University of Minnesota
Box 721-UMHC
Harvard Street at East River Road
Minneapolis, MN 55455
NCYD is an information and resource center focusing on adolescents with chronic illnesses and disabilities and the issues surrounding their transition to adult life.

National Clearinghouse on Family Support and Children's Mental Health
Portland State University
PO Box 751
Portland, OR 97207
(503) 725-4040
1-800-628-1696

National Council on Disability (NCD)*
800 Independence Ave., SW
Washington, DC 20591
(202) 267-3846
The purpose of this council is to promote policies, programs, practices, and procedures that guarantee equal opportunity to all individuals with disabilities regardless of the nature or severity of the disability; and to empower individuals with disabilities to achieve economic self-sufficiency, independent living, and inclusion and integration into all aspects of society.

National Health Information Center (ONHIC)*
PO Box 1133
Washington, DC 20013-1133
(301) 565-4167
1-800-336-4797

National Maternal and Child Health Clearinghouse
38th and R Sts. NW
Washington, DC 20057
(202)625-8410
The clearinghouse distributes current publications on maternal
and child health and human genetic issues, including topics
such as pregnancy, nutrition, special health needs, chronic
illness, and disabilities.

National Easter Seal Society
70 East Lake St.
Chicago, IL 60601
(312) 726-6200
(312) 726-4258
1-800-221-6827
The National Easter Seal Society provides services that include comprehensive medical or vocational rehabilitation, technological assistance,
recreation, equipment loans, public education, advocacy, and programs
for the prevention and treatment of disabling conditions.

National Information Center for Children and Youth with Disabilities
(NICCYD)*
PO Box 1492
Washington, DC 20013
1-800-999-5599
NICCYD provides free information to assist parents, educators, care-
givers, advocates, and others in helping children and you with disabili-
ties become participating members of the community.
Publication: NICHCY News Digest

National Information Clearinghouse (NIC) on Infants with Disabilities
and Life-Threatening Conditions*
Center for Developmental Disabilities
University of South Carolina
Benson Building 1st Floor
Columbia, SC 29208
1-800-922-9234 ext. 201
1-800-922-1107 in South Carolina
Information specialists at the NIC respond to individual requests and
assist families in accessing services such as parent support and training,

advocacy, health care, financial resources, early intervention, child protective services, and legal and other information resources.

National Organization on Disability (NOD)
910 16th St., NW, Suite 600
Washington, DC 20006

Sick Kids (need) Involved People (SKIP)
990 2nd Ave., 2nd Floor
New York, NY 10022
(212) 421-9160
(212) 421-9161

Genetics

National Genetic Foundation
555 W. 57th Street
New York, NY 10010

Alliance of Genetic Support Groups
1001 22nd Street, NW Suite 800
Washington, DC 20037
1-800-336-GENE
A bridge between consumers and service providers and a coalition of voluntary genetic support groups, consumers and professionals. The Alliance serves as a forum for addressing the needs of individuals and families affected by genetic disorders from a national and cross disability perspective.

Regional Genetics Networks
Ten Regional Genetics Networks cover all 50 states, the District of Columbia, Puerto Rico, and the Virgin Islands, whose mission is to plan, implement and evaluate a program integrating genetic services into a comprehensive system of family centered, community-based care.

Genetics Network of the Empire State (GENES)*
NEW YORK
NYS Dept. of Health, WCL&R, Room E-275
PO Box 509
Albany, NY 12201-0509
(518) 474-7148
FAX: (518) 474-8590
Newsletter: GENESIS

Great Lakes Regional Genetics Group (GLaRGG)*
IN, IL, MI, MN, OH, WI
328 Waisman Center
1500 Highland Avenue
Madison, WI 53705-2280
(608) 265-2907
FAX: (608) 262-3496
Newsletter: Great Lakes Genetic News

Great Plains Genetics Service Network (GPGSN)*
AR, IA, KS, MO, NB, ND, OK, SD
University of Iowa, Dept. of Pediatrics
Division of Medical Genetics
Iowa City, IA 52241
(319) 356-2674
FAX: (319) 356-3347
Newsletter: Genexus

Mid-Atlantic Regional Human Genetics Network (MARHGN)*
DE, DC, MD, NJ, PA, VA, WV
Albert Einstein Medical Center, Korman Bldg.
5501 Old York Road - Room B-29
Philadelphia, PA 19141-3098
(215) 456-7910
FAX: (215) 456-7911
Newsletter: MARGIN

Mountain States Regional Genetic Services Network (MSRGSN)*
AZ, CO, MT, NM, UT, WY
Colorado Dept. of Health Family Health Service Div.
4210 East 11th Avenue
Denver, CO 80220
(303) 331-8376
FAX: (303) 320-1529
Newsletter: Genetic Drift

New England Regional Genetics Group (NERGG)*
CT, ME, MA, NH, RI, VT
PO Box 682
Gorham, ME 04038-0682
(207) 839-5324
FAX: (207) 839-8637
Newsletter: NERGG News in Genetic Resources

Pacific Northwest Regional Genetics Group (PacNoRGG)*
AK, ID, OR, WA
PO Box 574
Portland, OR 97207-0574
(503) 494-8342
FAX: (503) 494-4447
Newsletter: Genetics Northwest

Pacific Southwest Regional Genetics Network (PSRGN)*
CA, HI, NV
State of California Dept. of Health Services
Genetic Disease Branch
2151 Berkeley Way, Annex 4
(510) 540-2696
FAX: (510) 540-2966
Newsletter: Genetically Speaking

Southeastern Regional Genetics Group (SERGG)*
AL, FL, GA, KY, LA, MS, NC, SC, TN
Emory University School of Medicine
2040 Ridgewood Drive
Atlanta, GA 30322
(404)727-5844
FAX: (404)727-5783
Newsletter: SERGG

Texas Genetics Network (TEXGENE)*
TEXAS
Texas Dept. of Health
Bureau of Maternal and Child Health
100 West 49th Street
Austin, TX 78756-3199
(512) 458-7700
FAX: (512) 458-7421
Newsletter: TEXGENE

Growth Disorders

Human Growth Foundation
PO Box 3090
Falls Church, VA 22043
(800) 451-6434
Helping individuals and families affected by growth disorders through
national conferences, pamphlets, a monthly newsletter, and research
grants for studies of growth and growth disorders.

Little People of America
PO Box 9897
Washington, DC 20016
(301)589-0730
Provides information and conferences to people with various forms of
short stature.

Short Stature Foundation, Inc.
17200 Jamboree Road, Suite J
Irvine, CA 92714-5828
(714) 474-4554
FAX: (714)474-2145
Helpline: 1-800-24DWARF
Providing enhanced public awareness, and service, information and advocacy to enhance the positive well being and independence of short statured/dwarfed individuals.

Hearing Disorders

American Speech-Language-Hearing Assn. (ASHA)
10801 Rockville Pike
Rockville, MD 20852
(301) 897-5700
1-800-638-8255

Alexander Graham Bell Assoc. for the Deaf
3417 Volta, NW
Washington, DC 20007

The Better Hearing Institute
1430 K. Street, North, Suite 600
Washington, DC 20005

Boys Town National Research Hospital
555 N. 30th Street
Omaha, NE 68131-9909

National Association for the Deaf
814 Thayer Avenue
Silver Spring, MD 20910

National Information Center on Deafness*
Gallaudet University
800 Florida Avenue N.E.

Washington, DC 20002
(202) 651-5051
(202) 651-5052

Self Help for Hard of Hearing People (SHHH)
7800 Wisconsin Ave.
Bethesda, MD 20814
(800)301-657-2248

Legal Rights

Disability Rights Education and Defense Fund (DREDF)
2212 Sixth Street
Berkeley, CA 94710
(510) 644-2555
(510) 644-2629
DREDF is a national nonprofit organization run primarily by persons
with disabilities to achieve the goals of the disability rights movement.

National Association of Protection and Advocacy Systems (NAPS)
900 Second Street NE, Suite 211
Washington, DC 20002
(202) 408-9514
(202) 408-9521
The National Association of Protection and Advocacy System, Inc. is a
voluntary membership organization of state programs advocating for the
rights of people with developmental disabilities.

Library Services

National Library Service for the Blind & Physically Handicapped
The Library of Congress*
Washington, D.C. 20542
(202) 707-5100

National Library of Medicine
8600 Rockville Pike
Bethesda, MD 20894

Professional Organizations

American Occupational Therapy Association (AOTA)
1383 Piccard Drive, Suite 300
Rockville, MD 20850
1-800-336-9799

American Academy of Orthopaedic Surgeons
222 South Prospect Ave.
Park Ridge, IL 60068
1-800-346-AAOS

American Massage Therapy Association
1130 W. North Shore Ave.
Chicago, IL 60626

American Physical Therapy Association
1111 North Fairfax St.
Alexandria, VA 22314
(703) 684-2782

Shriners's Hospital Referral Line
1-800-237-5055
1-800-282-9161 (in Florida)
Free orthopaedic treatment for children under age 18

Rare Disorders

National Organization for Rare Disorders (NORD)
PO Box 8923
New Fairfield, CT 06812
(203) 746-6518
NORD provides information about thousands of rare disorders and
brings families with similar disorders together for mutual support. It
also promotes research, accumulates and disseminates
information about orphan drugs and devices, provides technical
assistance to newly organized support groups, and educates the general
public and medical professionals about diagnosis and treatment of rare
disorders.

Recreation and Leisure

Arts
PO Box 2040
Grand Central Station
New York, NY 10007

Music Services Unit
Library of Congress
Division for the Blind and Physically Handicapped
1201 16th Street, NW
Washington, DC 20542

American Association for Health, Physical Education and Recreation
Program for the Handicapped
1201 16th Street, NW
Washington, DC 20036

Rehabilitation

Association for the Advancement of Rehabilitation Technology (RESNA)
1101 Connecticut Ave. NW, Suite 700
Washington, DC 20036
(202) 857-1199

Independent Living Res. Utilization Project (ILRU)
The Institute for Rehabilitation and Research
3400 Bissonnet, Suite 101
Houston, TX 77005
(713) 666-6244

National Institute on Disability and Rehabilitation Research (NIDRR)
330 C Street SW
Washington, DC 20202
(202) 205-9151
(202) 205-9136
NIDRR provides leadership and support for a national and international
program of comprehensive and coordinated research on the rehabilitation of individuals with disabilities.

National Rehabilitation Information Center (NARIC/ABLEDATA)*
8455 Colesville Road, Suite 935
Silver Spring, MD 20910-3319
1-800- 346-2742
The NARIC is a library and information center on disability and rehabilitation.

Service Dogs

Assistance Dogs of America
8806 State Route 64
Swanton, Ohio 43558
(419) 825-3622

Canine Companions for Independence
National Office
4350 Occidental Rd.
PO Box 446
Santa Rosa, CA 95402-0446
(707) 528-0830

Canine Partners for Life
130D, RD2
Cochranville, PA 19330
(215) 869-4902

New England Assistance Dog Service (NEADS)
PO Box 213
West Boylston, MA 01583
(508) 835-3304

Paws with A Cause
1235 100th Street, S.E.
Byron Center, MI 49315
(616)698-0688

Sexuality

Sex Information and Education Council of the United States (SIECUS)
130 West 42nd Street, Suite 2500
New York, NY 10036
(212) 819-9770

Support for Parents and Families

Access/Abilities
PO Box 458
Mill Valley, CA 94942
(415) 388-3250
Access/Abilities is a consulting, problem solving firm dedicated to
finding resources for a better life beyond functionality and independence.

Beach Center on Families and Disability
University of Kansas
3111 Haworth Hall
Lawrence, KS 66045
(913) 864-7607
This national directory describes services provided, available materials,
program demographics, and families and disabilities served by
programs throughout the United States. Local Parent-to-Parent
Programs are in every state.

CAPP National Parent Resource Center
Federation for Children with Special Needs
95 Berkeley Street, Suite 104
Boston, MA 02116
(617) 482-2915
1-800-331-0688
This organization is a parent-run resource system designed to further
the goals of family-centered, community-based, comprehensive, and
coordinated systems of health care for children with special needs and
their families.

Family Resource Center on Disabilities
20 East Jackson Boulevard, Room 900
Chicago, IL 60604
1-800-952-4199
(312) 939-3513
(312) 939-3519
The Family Resource Center on Disabilities is a coalition of parent and professional organizations that educates and trains parents and professionals on special education rights.

National Parent Network on Disabilities (NPND)
1600 Prince Street, Suite 115
Alexandria, VA 22314
(703) 684-6763
NPND'S mission is to speak as the collective voice representing the perspectives, needs, and interests of parents and family members of persons of all ages with a disability, regardless of the type of disability.
Parent Care
9041 Colgate Street
Indianapolis, IN 46268-1210
(317) 872-9913
Parent Care is a national focal point for information, referral, and support for families of infants who require special care at birth.

Parents Helping Parents: The Parent-Directed Family Resource Center for Children with Special Needs
535 Race Street, Suite 140
San Jose, CA 95126
(408) 288-5010
Parents Helping Parents provides information, such as a library, newsletter, resources, and referrals; support including parent-to-parent matches, sibling fun days, and over 20 specialty
groups; and training on individual education programs (IEPs) and supplemental security income.

Sibling Information Network
CT University Affiliated Program
991 Main St., Suite 3A
East Hartford, CT 06108
(203) 282-7050

Technical Assistance to Parent Programs (TAPP) Network
National Office
Federation for Children with Special Needs
95 Berkeley Street, Suite 104
Boston, MA 02116
(617) 482-2915

Travel

Accessible Adventure, Inc.
1050 Browlee Rd.
PO Box 16137
Memphis, TN 38116
(901) 385-2718

Flying Wheels
143 West Bridge Street
Box 382
Owatonna, MD 55060
(800) 533-0363

Whole Person Tours
PO Box 1084
Bayonne, NJ 07002
(201) 858-3400

Wings on Wheels Tours
Evergreen Travel Tours Service
19505 44th Avenue West
Lynwood, WA 98036
(206) 776-1184

Some federally funded resources are marked with an (*).

Catalogues of Interest to People with Osteogenesis Imperfecta

Aids for Independent Living

Enrichments
PO Box 471
Western Springs, IL 60558-0471
1-800-323-5547
Extensive collection of adaptive devices.

OIF Adaptive Equipment & Reference Manual
The Osteogenesis Imperfecta Foundation, Inc.
5505 W. Laurel St., Suite 210
Tampa, FL 33607
(813) 282-1161
A collection of equipment and resources, resulting from many requests for items found to be specifically recommended or utilized by people with OI and/or their caregivers.
(Contributions toward printing costs are requested.)

Clothing

Avenues Unlimited
1199 Avenida ACASO/ Suite K
Camarillo, CA 93012
1-800-848-2837 Customer Service Line
A wide variety of clothing for wheelchair users. Many of the small sizes could be altered for small stature individuals.

Child's Play
3359 Collingwood SW
Wyoming, MI 49509
(616) 530-2471
Custom sewn adaptive clothing for children and young adults at reasonable prices.

Exceptionally Yours
Box 3246
Framington, MA 01701
(508) 877-9757
Children's and young adult sizes in adapted casual clothing

Freedom Designs
PO Box 528179
Port Clinton, OH 43452
(419) 635-2256
Wheelchair fashions

On The Rise
2282 Four Oaks Grange Road
Eugene, OR 97405

Cinderella of Boston
PO Box 7110
Canoga Park, CA 91304
Women's shoes in small sizes

Cole-Haan
North Elm Street
Yearmouth, MA 04096-5002
Men's shoes in small sizes

Medical and Home Health Supplies

Abbey Medical
13782 Crenshaw Blvd.
Gardena, CA 90249

Fred Sammons, Inc.
145 Tower Drive
Burr Ridge, IL 60521
(800) 323-5547
Ask to receive their Professional Healthcare Catalogue and information
about their "Be OK Self-Help Aids". Full of equipment and supplies.

J.A. Preston Corporation
71 Fifth Ave.
New York, NY 10003

Recreation

ABLEDATA*
1-800-346-2742
1-800-447-4221 (Illinois residents)
Free service providing information about over 25,000 different pieces of adaptive equipment.

Access to Recreation
2509 E. Thousand Oaks Blvd., Suite 430
Thousand Oaks, CA 91362

Danmar Products, Inc.
221 Jackson Industrial Drive
Ann Arbor, MI 48103
Specializes in swim aids for adapted aquatics.

Magic In Motion
20604 84th Ave. South
Kent, WA 98032
Supplier of Cycle-One hand-pedalled wheelchair attachment.

J.L. Pachner, Ltd.
13 Via Nola
Laguna Niguel, CA 92577
Specializes in products to assist the disabled sportsman, including fishing aids.

Rehabilitation

National Rehabilitation Information Center (NARIC)
8455 Colesville Road Suite 935
Silver Springs, MD 20910
1-800-346-2742
1-800-227-0216
(301) 588-9284

Splinting and First Aid Supplies

Jobst
Box 653
Toledo, OH 43694
(419) 698-1611
Manufactures the EMTech Vacuum Splint, which converts from soft to rigid in seconds. Conforms to the limb providing immobilization and support.

W.L. Gore and Associates, Inc.
Flagstaff, AZ
The Gortex Cast Liner provides a waterproof liner inside a cast. The Gortex Liner allows the wearer to shower and bath without covering the cast.

Toys

Consumer Care Products
PO Box 684
Sheboygan, WI 53082-0684
(414) 459-8353
Scooter boards, cycles, and other equipment

Enabling Devices
A Division of Toys for Special Children
385 Warburton Avenue
Hastings-on-Hudson, NY 10706
Environmental controls, switches and adaption, and switch toys

Equipment Shop
Box 33
Bedford, MA 01730
(617) 275-7681
Carries the PORT A Play and other recreational equipment

Flaghouse, Inc.
150 N. MacQuesten Pkwy.
Mt. Vernon, NY 10550
(914) 699-1900

H.O.P.E./T.M.
Innovative Products Inc.
830 S. 48th Street
Grand Fork, ND 58201
(800) 950-5185
(701)772-5185
Motorizes toy trucks

Pocket Full of Therapy
PO Box 174
Morganville, NJ 07751
(908) 290-0711
A number of fun things

Rifton
PO Box 901
Rifton, NY 12471-0901
(800) 374-3866
Rock N' Roll Machines
3405 69th Drive
Lubbock, TX 79413
(800) 654-9664
Sturdy three wheel cycles

The Right Start Catalog
Right Start Plaza
Westlake Village, CA 91361-4627
Good selection of toys and equipment for infants and young
children.

Appendix E

Recommended Reading

Books and Videos

Aids and Adapted Equipment

Caston, Don. *Easy to Make Aids for your Handicapped Child: A Guide for Parents and Teachers.* Englewood Cliffs, NJ: Prentice-Hall, 1981.

Levin, Jackie, M.S. and Lynn Scherfenberg, R.P.T. *Selection and Use of Simple Technology - in Home, School Work, and the Community.* Available from the Special Needs Project, (800)333-6867. Very practical suggestions for switches and gadgets.

Resources in Special Education (RISE)
650 Howe Avenue, Suite 300
Sacramento, CA 95825
(916) 641-5925
(916) 894-9799
RISE develops and disseminates information and resources to professionals and parents involved in the education of children with disabilities.

Rural Institute on Disabilities
52 Corbin Hall
The University of Montana
Missoula, MT 59812
(406) 243-5467
1-800-732-0323
The Rural Institute of Disabilities promotes the full participation in rural life by individuals of all ages with disabilities by developing and disseminating innovations in teaching, research, community services, and policy advocacy.

Employment

Center on Education and Training for Employment
1900 Kenny Road
Columbus, OH 43210-1090
(614) 292-4353
The Mission of the Center on Education and Training for Employment is to facilitate the career and occupational preparation and advancement of youth and adults.

JAN (Job Accommodation Network)
West Virginia University
809 Allen Hall
PO Box 6123
Morgantown, WV 26506-6123
JAN brings together information from many sources about practical steps employers can take to make accommodations for the functional limitations of employees and applicants with disabilities.

Clothing

Kennedy, Evelyn S., *Dressing with Pride: Clothing Changes for Special Needs.* Groton, CT: Pride Foundation, 1981.

Education

Anderson, Winifred, Stephen Chitwood, and Deidre Hayden. *The Special Education Maze - A Guide for Parents and Teachers.* Available from the Special Needs Project, (800)333-6867.

Finding and Utilizing the Medical Help You Need

Bursztajn, Harold, M.D. et al. *Medical Choices, Medical Chances: How Patients, Families, and Physicians Can Cope with Uncertainty.* New York: Delta, 1983.

Gots, Ronald, M.D. and Arthur Kaufman, M.D. *The People's Hospital Book.* New York: Avon, 1978.

Winter, Arthur, M.D. and Ruth Winter. *Consumer's Guide to Free Medical Information by Phone and by Mail.* New Jersey: Prentice Hall, 1993.

Learning to Accept a Disability

Darling, Rosalyn B., and Jon. *Children Who Are Different.* St. Louis: C.V. Mosby Company, 1982.

Des Jardins, Charlotte. *How to Get Services by Being Assertive.* Chicago: Chicago Coordinating Council for Handicapped Children, 1990.

Krementz, Jill. *How It Feels To Live With A Physical Disability.* Simon & Shuster. Contains a chapter written by a teenaged girl who has OI. Very good for teens.

Kushner, Harold. *When Bad Things Happen to Good People.*, New York: Schocken, 1983.

Shapiro, Joseph. *No Pity - People With Disabilities Forging a New Civil Rights Movement.* Random House. Very enlightening reading - makes you think about disabilities in a whole new way.

Shields, C.V. Strategies: *A Practical Guide for Dealing with Professionals and Human Service Systems.* Richmond Hill, Ontario: Human Services Press, 1987.

Osteogenesis Imperfecta, Brittle Bones, and Short Stature

Scott, C., Mayeux, N. Crandall, R., *Dwarfism, The Family and Professional Guide,* Short Stature Foundation, Irvine, CA. 1994. Available by calling (800) 24-DWARF.

Kanga, I. *Trying to Grow.* Picador, 1990.

Kenihan, Kerry. *Quentin.* Available from the Special Needs Project, (800)333-6867. Young boy with OI and the founding of the Australian OI Foundation.

The OI Newborn - A Loving Look at the Future, (30 min. video) Available through: The Osteogenesis Imperfecta Foundation, Inc., 5005 W. Laurel St. Suite 210, Tampa, FL 33632, (813)282-1161.

Within Reach, (50 min. video) Looks at examples of people with osteogenesis imperfecta who have either achieved or who are working toward independent living. Available through: The Osteogenesis Imperfecta Foundation, Inc., 5005 W. Laurel St. Suite 210, Tampa, FL 33632, (813)282-1161.

Look How Far We've Come, (13 min. video) An introduction to osteogenesis imperfecta and the Osteogenesis Imperfecta Foundation. The video highlights the spirit and accomplishments of Foundation volunteers over the past years. (1990) Available through: The Osteogenesis Imperfecta Foundation, Inc., 5005 W. Laurel St. Suite 210, Tampa, FL 33632, (813)282-1161.

Peck, William, M.D. and Louis Aviolo, M.D., *Osteoporosis: The Silent Thief.* Washington, DC: American Association of retired Persons.

Teens, Independent Living, and Preparing for the Future

Feingold, S. Norman and Norma R. Miller. *Your Future: A Guide for the Handicapped Teenager.* New York: Richards Rosen Press,1981.

Russell, L. Mark. *A Family Guide to Legal and Financial Planning for the Disabled.* Evanston, IL: First Publications, 1983.

Swirnoff, Weinberg, and Daly. *Planning for the Disabled Child.* Minneapolis: Northwestern Mutual Life Insurance Company (free publication).

Sexuality

Brookes, Paul H. *Disability, Sexuality, and Abuse: An Annotated Bibliography.* Baltimore, MD 1991. More than 1,100 entries.

Sports and Recreation

American Academy of Orthopaedic Surgeons, sponsor. *Sports and Recreational Programs for the Child and Young Adult with Physical Disability.* Proceedings of the Winter Park Seminar, Chicago, IL, April 11-13, 1983.

Support for Parents and Families

Biklen, Douglas. *Let Our Children Go.* Syracuse: Human Policy Press, 1974.

Buscaglia, Leo, ed. *The Disabled and Their Parents.* New York: Holt, Rinehart, and Winston, 1983.

Featherstone, Helen. *A Difference in the Family,* New York: Penguin, 1981.

Finston, Peggy, M.D. *Parenting Plus - Raising Children with Special Health Needs.* Available from the Special Needs Project, (800)333-6867. Discusses emotional aspects of raising children with special needs and giving the child some choice in their care.

McCollum, Audry T. *The Chronically Ill Child: A Guide for Parents and Professionals.* New Haven: Yale University Press, 1981.

Meyer, D.J., Vadasy, P., and Fewell, R. *Living with a Brother or Sister with Special Needs.* Seattle: University of Washington Ress, 1985.

Moore, Cory. *Reader's Guide for Parents of Children with Mental, Physical, or Emotional Disabilities.* Rockville, MD: Woodbine House, 1990. Comprehensive listing of books, articles, films, videos.

National Library Service for the Blind and Physically Handicapped. *Selected Readings for Parents of Handicapped Children: A Bibliography.* Washington, DC 20542: Library of Congress

Schmitt, Christopher. *Parent Resource Directory for Parents and Professionals Caring for Children with Chronic Illness or Disabilities.* Bethesda, MD: Association for the Care of Children's Health, 1991. Names, addresses, and phone numbers of U.S. and Canadian parent/counselors with their expertise on specific disabilities.

Simons, Robin. *After the Tears - Parents Talk About Raising A Child With A Disability.* New York: Harcourt Brace Jovanovich, 1987. Available from the Special Needs Project, (800)333-6867. This is an excellent book for new parents.

Sullivan, Tom. *Special Parent, Special Child.* G. P. Putman's Sons, NY, 1995. Discusses children's disabilities from the parents' perspective and stresses the importance of parent advocacy. Excellent book for parents of the very yound.

Sullivan, Tom. *If You Could See What I Hear.* G. P. Putnam's Sons, NY, 1991. Excellent – discusses growing up blind. Information applicable to all disabilities.

Turnbull, A. P. and H. R. *Parents Speak Out: Then and Now.* Columbus, OH: Charles Merrill, 1985.

Travel

Weiss, L., *Access to the World,* Owl Books, Henry Holt, 1986. Detailed information on accessibility to 14 chain hotels as well as details on menus and special arrangements for special travel.

Barish, F., *Frommer's A Guide for the Disabled Traveler*, Frommer/Pasmantier, 1984. Designed for wheelchair travelers and others with mobility limitations. Detailed accessibility on 15 major cities in the U.S., Canada, and Europe.

The Handicapped Driver's Mobility Guide, American Automobile Association, 1984. Free to AAA members. Traffic Safety Department, 8111 Gatehouse Rd., Falls Church, VA 22047.
Lists companies and services for specialized driving equipment and information of special driver training.

Newsletters and Magazines

Accent on Living
Accent on Information, Inc.
PO Box 700
Bloomington, IL 61701

Better Health Care for Less Newsletter
Better Health Care for Less
PO Box 15369
Atlanta, GA 30333
(404) 816-6548

Exceptional Parent
1170 Commonwealth Avenue, 3rd floor
Boston, MA 02134-4646.
Not just a magazine - virtually a parent support network.
Published eight times a year.

For Sibs Only (ages 4-9)
Sibling Forum (ages 10 and up)
Family Resource Association, Inc.
35 Haddon Ave.
Shrewsbury, NJ 07701

Kaleidoscope: International Magazine of Literature, Fine Arts, and Disability.
326 Locust Street
Akron, OH 44302-1876

Report from Closer Look
Closer Look
National Information Center for the Handicapped
PO Box 1492
Washington, DC 20013

Handy-Cap Horizons
Handy-Cap Horizons
3250 East Loretta Drive
Indianapolis, IN 46227

National Hookup
Indoor Sports Club
1145 Highland Street
Napoleon, OH 42545

NAPH National Newsletter
National Association of the Physically Handicapped
6473 Grandville Avenue
Detroit, MI 49229

Report
National Center for a Barrier-Free Environment
8401 Connecticut Ave.
Washington, DC 20036

National Wheelchair Athletic Association Newsletter
National Wheelchair Athletic Association
40-24 62nd Street
Woodside, NY 1370

Challenge Magazine
2117 Buffalo Road, Suite 254
Rochester, NY 14624
Free subscription.
Addresses issues of disabled persons.

Appendix F

Healthy Eating for Children with OI

Figure 4-1

A Guide for Feeding Children of Different Ages*

Food	Servings per day	Average Serving Size					Comments
		1 year	2-3 years	4-5 years	6-9 years	10-12 years	
Milk & Dairy Products	4	½ cup	½-¾ cup	¾ cup	¾-1 cup	1 cup	Substitutions for 1 C. milk: 1.5 oz cheese, 1 cup yogurt
Meat group Lean meat, fish, poultry, or equivalent	2-3	½ - 1 oz.	1 oz.	2 oz.	2-4 oz.	3-4 oz	Substitutions for 1 oz. meat or poultry: 1 egg, 2 T. peanut butter, ¼ - ⅓ C. cooked legumes
Fruits & Vegetables	5 - 9						
Vitamin C source	1 or more	⅓ cup	½ cup	½ cup	½ cup	½ cup	- Includes 1 vitamin C-rich fruit, vegetable or juice.
Vitamin A source	1 or more	2 Tbsp	3 Tbsp	¼ cup	¼ cup	⅓ cup	- Includes one green leafy or yellow vegetable or fruit.
Other vegetables & fruits	3 or more	2 Tbsp	3 Tbsp	¼ cup	⅓ cup	½ cup	
Breads & Cereals:	6 - 11						
Whole grain or enriched bread		½ slice	½ - 1 slice	1-1½ slice	1-1½ slice	1 - 2 slices	
Ready to eat cereal		2 Tbsp	¼ - ⅓ cup	⅓ - ½ cup	½ - ¾ cup	¾ - 1 cup	
Cooked cereals, (including macaroni, rice, etc.)		2 Tbsp	¼ - ⅓ cup	⅓ - ½ cup	½ cup	¾ cup	

* Adapted from Lucus, B.: *Nutrition in Childhood.* In Mahan, L.K. and Arlin, M.: *Krause's Food Nutrition & Diet Therapy,* 8th Edition, Philadelphia, W.B. Saunders Company, 1992, and *The Food Guide Pyramid,* USDA, Human Nutrition Info. Service.